SpringerBriefs in Psychology

SpringerBriefs present concise summaries of cutting-edge research and practical applications across a wide spectrum of fields. Featuring compact volumes of 55 to 125 pages, the series covers a range of content from professional to academic. Typical topics might include:

- A timely report of state-of-the-art analytical techniques
- A bridge between new research results as published in journal articles and a contextual literature review
- A snapshot of a hot or emerging topic
- An in-depth case study or clinical example
- A presentation of core concepts that readers must understand to make independent contributions

SpringerBriefs in Psychology showcase emerging theory, empirical research, and practical application in a wide variety of topics in psychology and related fields. Briefs are characterized by fast, global electronic dissemination, standard publishing contracts, standardized manuscript preparation and formatting guidelines, and expedited production schedules.

Maor Katz • Michael J. Christensen
Alexandre Vaz • Tony Rousmaniere

Deliberate Practice of TEAM-CBT

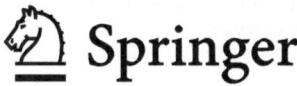 Springer

Maor Katz
Director and Founder
Feeling Good Institute
Mountain View, CA, USA

Michael J. Christensen
Director of Professional Development
Feeling Good Institute
Mountain View, CA, USA

Alexandre Vaz
Director of Training
Sentio University
Los Angeles, CA, USA

Tony Rousmaniere
President
Sentio University
Los Angeles, CA, USA

ISSN 2192-8363   ISSN 2192-8371   (electronic)
SpringerBriefs in Psychology

ISBN 978-3-031-46018-0   ISBN 978-3-031-46019-7   (eBook)
https://doi.org/10.1007/978-3-031-46019-7

This Springer imprint is published by the registered company Springer Nature Switzerland AG
The registered company address is: Gewerbestrasse 11, 6330 Cham, Switzerland

Paper in this product is recyclable.

Acknowledgments

Maor and Mike would like to acknowledge Dr. David Burns for his brilliance and generosity in developing and teaching TEAM-CBT. His incredible gift of training and mentoring is unmatched and we are deeply grateful for the ways he has inspired, challenged, and encouraged us personally in our learning journey.

We would like to express our heartfelt thanks to all of our colleagues at the Feeling Good Institute who share in our passion for delivering exceptional therapy and strive to provide world-class training to facilitate it. A special thanks to the following supervisors and trainees who tested exercises and/or provided invaluable feedback on the DP exercises presented in this book:

Jennelle, Michelle, Barbara, Brad, Dan, Amber, Brian, Lorna, Kate, Heather, Mor, Noelle, Joanna, Suzanne, Kristina, Hollie, Anastasia, Pedro, Peter, Kamila, Steve, LJ, Jill, Angela, and Taylor.

A special thank you to Kevin Pillsbury who graciously offered to share his inspiring experience in a live TEAM CBT therapy session. We would also like to acknowledge Dr. Heather Clague who demonstrated her masterful skills as co-therapist with Mike in the live therapy demonstration.

Our families have, and continue to be, our greatest source of support and encouragement. They have sacrificed much in giving us freedom to pursue this project. We love you and appreciate all you do for us.

Contents

About the Authors

Maor Katz, MD, completed his medical studies at the Hadassah-Hebrew University Medical School in Jerusalem. He continued as a postdoctoral scholar at Stanford University School of Medicine where he trained extensively with Dr. David Burns. Dr. Katz serves on the adjunct faculty at Stanford University Department of Psychiatry and Behavioral Sciences. He has many publications in the field of depression, anxiety, and resilience and has won several teaching and research awards. In 2013, Dr. Katz founded the Feeling Good Institute, a center with a worldwide reach, dedicated to helping therapists become more effective through training and treatment in TEAM-CBT.

Mike Christensen, MA, is Director of Professional Development at the Feeling Good Institute. He is cofounder of the Feeling Good Institute Canada and serves as its Clinical Director. Mr. Christensen is a Level 5 TEAM CBT Master Therapist and Trainer and provides advanced level online and in person training at workshops, webinars, and seminars around the world. His diverse background in business, leadership, theology, and as an elite-level athlete has served to enhance his unique skill set as a therapist, communicator, teacher, and trainer.

Alexandre Vaz, PhD, is cofounder and Chief Academic Officer of Sentio University and the Sentio Counseling Center. He provides workshops, webinars, and advanced clinical training and supervision to clinicians around the world. Dr. Vaz is the author/co-editor of over a dozen books on deliberate practice and psychotherapy training. He has held multiple committee roles for the Society for the Exploration of Psychotherapy Integration (SEPI) and the Society for Psychotherapy Research (SPR). Dr. Vaz is founder and host of "Psychotherapy Expert Talks," an acclaimed interview series with distinguished psychotherapists and therapy researchers.

Tony Rousmaniere, PsyD, is cofounder and Program Director of Sentio University and the Sentio Counseling Center. He provides workshops, webinars, and advanced clinical training and supervision to clinicians around the world. Dr. Rousmaniere is the author/co-editor of over a dozen books on deliberate practice and psychotherapy training. In 2017, he published the widely cited article in *The Atlantic Monthly*, "What your therapist doesn't know." Dr. Rousmaniere supports the open-data movement and publishes his aggregated clinical outcome data, in de-identified form, on his website at www.drtonyr.com. Dr. Rousmaniere is President-Elect of Division 29 of the American Psychological Association (Society for the Advancement of Psychotherapy).

Part I
Theory and Concepts

Chapter 1
TEAM-CBT and Deliberate Practice

Overview of TEAM-CBT

When I (M.K.) entered the small conference room at the Stanford Department of Psychiatry and was greeted by David Burns for the first time, I did not yet know that he was a superstar. I was most impressed by his warm welcome and his shocking pink Hawaiian shirt. Ten minutes later, I realized that I had found myself in a place of wonder. In this room was exactly the kind of therapy I wanted to practice: warm, connected, humble, at eye level, and at the same time ruthless. Doing whatever it takes to overcome suffering, with both patients and therapists held accountable and to high standards. It was not yet called TEAM-CBT, it was just therapy.

This was 2005, and David had been teaching his psychotherapy seminar for a few years by then, but there were only eight people in attendance. Five years later, the "Tuesday Group" was so large that it had to be moved to the largest conference room in the building and divided into two with me leading the "Wednesday Group" for "newbies." Since then, TEAM-CBT took off with a super successful podcast that was listened to by millions, and therapists all over the world train it and become trainers themselves in the approach.

Dr. Burns is best known for his seminal book *Feeling Good, The New Mood Therapy*, published in 1980, which made cognitive therapy accessible to the general public and is one of the most successful self-help books of all time, having sold many millions of copies worldwide. Dr. Burns published several other self-help books (Burns, 1980, 1993, 1999, 2010). However, David's brilliant approach to training therapists is less well known (Burns, 1997). Until recently, this work was mostly available to those lucky few who happened upon his Stanford Tuesday Group.

TEAM-CBT provides a road map for therapists on how to provide therapy that works. It views the therapist as a continuously improving professional, who needs help and opportunities to practice, receive feedback, and try again. It is a transdiagnostic approach that identifies the inevitable stuck points in therapy and teaches

M. Katz et al., *Deliberate Practice of TEAM-CBT*, SpringerBriefs in Psychology, https://doi.org/10.1007/978-3-031-46019-7_1

therapists a set of skills on how to navigate the patient through them and move forward.

TEAM-CBT maps out therapy as a predictable path of discovery, confronting obstacles and reaching therapy goals. Therapists have four sets of skills to internalize and use sequentially:

T – Testing: Collecting and reviewing mood scores and other measures at every session.

E – Empathy: Focus on improving therapists' empathy and communication skills.

A – Agenda Setting/Assessment of Resistance: Five sequential steps to melt away resistance and boost motivation.

M – Methods: Rooted in CBT, while also drawing from a variety of modalities and schools of therapy, we use dozens of techniques to help our patients confront their negative thoughts and symptoms head-on. But only after we have addressed and honored resistance.

That is it! Get good at these four simple sets of skills and you will be a great therapist, guaranteed. However, it takes years to internalize and implement this well. It is challenging because, in the heat of the moment, in the therapy room, these skills suddenly become counterintuitive and anxiety provoking to us. Patients are never eager to fill out forms. Setting that expectation from patients and insisting that surveys be filled every session is hard for therapists to do. When it comes to empathy, we like to think we are naturally good at it. That is why we chose this profession in the first place. People experience us as easy to talk to, they confide in us, and find us to be good listeners. It is humbling to accept that we repeatedly and frequently fail at this most basic task of therapy: empathy. But once we accept our shortcomings, that is when we start improving.

The hardest skill set to internalize is the resistance-busting skill set. In TEAM-CBT, we view resistance as 100% expected and always there. However, it can be melted away if brought to our patients' conscious awareness. Dr. Burns often says that the greatest problem therapists have is that when patients ask for our help, we try to help them. It is because of our efforts and need to help that we create and maintain their resistance to change. I sometimes feel like I need nerves of steel to work well with a patient's resistance. To help people see what is good and beautiful about their symptoms and ask them to convince me that it is a good idea to overcome them. As a therapist, it is especially hard to advocate for the beauty and moral values of symptoms such as drug use, self-harm, procrastination, or hopelessness. Ultimately, our goal is to honor these symptoms, which provides the opportunity for the patient to be in charge of the direction of therapy and become the driving force in arguing for change. They become the ones convincing us rather than us, as therapists, trying to convince and motivate them. As a TEAM-CBT therapist, you will find yourself quickly doing all of that.

Until I learned TEAM-CBT, I was embarrassed to say that my patients' therapy process was meandering and reactive. I am Reactive because I was mostly trained as a therapist to respond to individual statements and problems that the patient poses. And meandering because it followed no clear overall path. A typical session would be a continuous series of patient statements responded to by me with no clear direction. All the while, I trusted that as long as I stayed the course long enough and trusted the process, it would lead to the patient feeling better.

The TEAM-CBT Road Map

Over the past decades, a significant body of research into therapy effectiveness has resulted in a much better understanding of the key factors for better outcomes in therapy. These include using routine outcome measurement in the therapy process (Boswell et al., 2015; Lambert et al., 2018; Persons et al. 2016; Solstad et al., 2021), therapists' ability to form therapeutic alliances (Howick et al., 2018; Huppert et al., 2014; Zilcha-Mano et al., 2016), patient-centered motivational approaches (Aviram et al., 2016; Burns et al., 2013; Pombo et al., 2016; Westra et al., 2016; Westra & Norouzian, 2018), and CBT methods (Angelakis et al., 2022; Boswell et al., 2013; Carpenter et al., 2018; Craske et al., 2014; Fang et al., 2013; Lungu et al., 2020). More recently, transdiagnostic, process-oriented approaches have started to emerge, helping therapists choose techniques more likely to help a particular patient (Hayes & Hofmann, 2018).

TEAM-CBT provides a simple, transdiagnostic road map for therapists to guide patients through the process of therapy, so it is no longer meandering and reactive, but rather goal oriented and focused. It weaves into the process many of those factors found through research to help therapy become more effective and makes it relatively easily accessible for therapists to learn, internalize, and integrate into their practice. It includes routine outcome measurement (Testing), improving therapists' therapeutic alliance (Empathy), motivational techniques to help patients become aware of their resistance to change and accountable to their own healing (Agenda Setting/Assessment of Resistance), and then use a myriad of CBT techniques in a playful and powerful way to finish the job (Methods). Together, it gives therapists a framework for better therapy and a workflow system that allows us to identify at any moment where we are on the map and gently guide our patients toward the next step in their recovery (Fig. 1.1).

The TEAM-CBT road map gives structure to each therapy session and to the therapy work as a whole. Every therapeutic encounter follows a flexible but sequential step-by-step approach that starts with a patient's self-measurement of symptoms (Testing), used not only to collect data but also to connect with the patient immediately at the start of the session at an emotional level (Empathy). With emphasis on

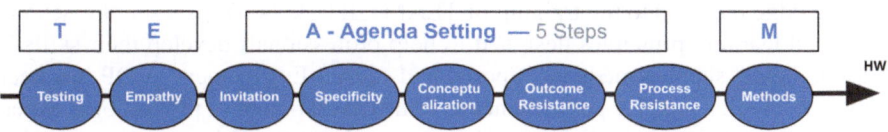

Fig. 1.1 The TEAM-CBT Workflow

empathy and compassion, the therapist moves through a process of focus on a specific challenge of the patient's choice (Invitation, Specificity), predicting the patient's likely themes of resistance to change and the work involved to achieve it (Conceptualization), then a counterintuitive focus on the good reasons not to overcome the challenge (Outcome Resistance), followed by the uncomfortable task of putting the responsibility for the work necessary for change squarely on the patient's shoulders (Process Resistance). After these steps are completed and the therapist is convinced that the patient is aware of the reasons not to change and committed to the work necessary for change, the therapist chooses with the patient techniques to help them confront their demons directly and achieve these goals (Methods).

When TEAM-CBT is done well, it has a certain rhythm to it as one progresses through the sequential steps: Testing – Empathy – Invitation – Specificity – Conceptualization – Outcome Resistance – Process Resistance – Methods – Testing, and repeat with the next goal.

The approach is simple to understand, fun, and straightforward, but difficult to implement.

The good news is that the TEAM-CBT road map for therapy not only gives therapists guidance on the next step and on the technique to be used at any time but also maps out where therapists are likely to feel challenged in taking the steps necessary to moving forward. Part of what the therapists love about TEAM-CBT is that it takes the complex process of therapy and makes it simple and easy to understand.

If you find it easy to expect more of your patients; to have them fill out mood scales before and after every session; to provide empathy and unconditional positive regard with no defensiveness or advice, even in the face of the most angry, hopeless, or inappropriate patient, all the while also sharing how you are truly feeling in a helpful way; to side with your patients' most upsetting symptoms and negative thoughts and feelings; and to expect your patients to do work outside of the therapy room and hold them accountable to it, then maybe this book is not for you. However, if any of those seem at least a little bit challenging for you, then you will find this book helpful and the approach refreshing. Every exercise in this book is designed to help you overcome your anxiety and discomfort in taking the necessary step in real time and to implement this powerful and humbling approach.

What Is Deliberate Practice?

This book uses the evidence-based training methods of deliberate practice (DP) to reliably increase the acquisition of clinical skills. We are excited to bring these cutting-edge methods to the training of TEAM CBT skills. DP is a set of research-informed learning principles designed to help professionals develop their skills in various fields, such as medicine, sports, and music. Engagement in DP has been shown to predict superior performance and the development of professional expertise over time (Ericsson et al., 2018). Here is how K. Anders Ericsson, the researcher who coined the term DP, summarized these learning principles:

Analyzing a review of laboratory studies of learning and skill acquisition during the last century, we found that improvement of performance was uniformly observed when people were given tasks with well-defined goals, were provided with feedback, and had ample opportunities for repetition. These deliberate efforts to increase one's performance beyond its current level involve problem solving and finding better methods to perform the tasks. When a person engages in a practice activity (typically designed by teachers) with the primary goal of improving some aspect of performance, we call that activity deliberate practice. (Ericsson, 2003, p. 67)

Vaz and Rousmaniere (2021, p. 22) summarized three key points from the accumulated DP research:

1. Top performers from different fields tend to maintain a DP training routine throughout their careers. This routine is usually composed of an individualized assessment of one's current performance and skill deficits, the establishment of well-defined learning goals, and a tailored plan focused on incremental skill development.
2. The DP regime should be constructed and supervised by a supervisor or trainer, who provides ongoing monitoring of skills and outcomes, and expert feedback on performance and practice.
3. DP occurs outside of one's comfort zone. It involves repeatedly engaging in tasks that are slightly beyond our current abilities (i.e., the "zone of proximal development"). It is also *deliberate*, in that it requires one's full attention, intention, and conscious actions. It is not enough to mechanically follow instructions from a trainer. Therefore, DP is a demanding, effortful activity that is usually neither easy nor enjoyable to sustain.

DP contrasts with and augments traditional training methods in several ways. Traditional learning methods often focus on passive methods such as reading and hearing lectures, while DP focuses on the more procedural and behavioral components that promote state-dependent learning (Ericsson & Pool, 2016). It focuses on direct observation and monitoring of one's work performance, provision of ongoing expert feedback from a trainer, and tailored behavioral rehearsal aimed at increasing one's performance (Ericsson & Pool, 2016; Rousmaniere et al., 2017). Research shows that these procedural learning methods are reliably more effective than passive methods at changing behavior (McGaghie et al., 2011; Cross et al., 2011; Beidas & Kendall, 2010; Beidas et al., 2014; Herschell et al., 2010). Interestingly, prominent mental health authors have argued that clinical training should include a procedural component. For example, in the field of psychotherapy, Safran and Muran (2000) wrote,

Training needs to go beyond the didactic presentation of declarative knowledge if therapists are going to develop the combination of procedural knowledge, self-awareness, and reflection-in-action skill necessary to respond to patients in a flexible and creative way. It is important for therapist training to include a substantial experiential component and to emphasize the process of personal growth. (pp. 206)

It is also noteworthy that mental health trainees consistently report that hands-on *practice* is the most helpful component of their skills training (Hill & Knox, 2013).

Despite these findings, many clinical trainings continue to emphasize passive and unsystematic learning methods (Hill & Knox, 2013), which is unfortunate given that, as Lambert and Ogles (1997) argue,

> If a mental health training program values the development of basic interpersonal or interviewing skills, this can best be achieved with a program that clearly specifies the skills to be learned and then develops training (including modeling and practice) directed at this goal. (p. 427)

Another distinctive feature of DP is its use of simulation-based mastery learning (SBML; Ericsson & Pool, 2016; Rousmaniere, 2016). These are "devices, trained persons, lifelike virtual environments, and contrived social situations that mimic problems, events, or conditions that arise in professional encounters" (McGaghie et al., 2014, p. 375). Simulation-based methods help professionals acquire skills by training in contexts that resemble those presented in real-life work performance. These methods provide the opportunity to practice and experiment with skills in the face of increasingly more challenging stimuli, which gradually enhances the professional's ability to perform effectively under stress. Anders Ericsson wrote of SBML as a core component of DP:

> Unlike surgery with actual patients, practice in the simulator can be stopped at any time, allowing trainees an immediate chance to correct mistakes and even repeatedly perform challenging parts of procedures … simulators offer the possibility of presenting rare problems and emergencies that would better prepare performers to deal with such situations. A recent study of military pilots showed that those pilots who had trained for a specific emergency situation in a simulator were more effective at responding to the same situation when it occurred during an actual flight mission. Similarly, surgeons who can experience rare emergency procedures when they are mentally ready in the simulator will be able to make necessary adjustments through additional training. These learning experiences are likely to better prepare surgeons for rare and challenging situations that occur unexpectedly. (Ericsson, 2004, p. S78)

For the DP of clinical skills, mental health professionals should use any form of simulation-based method that closely resembles actual clinical performance, such as the roleplaying of standardized patient statements portraying common clinical challenges. DP of clinical skills requires a balance between repetition and novelty, in that trainees should be repeatedly exposed to the same stimuli for behavioral rehearsal, while also being presented with new stimuli so they can experiment using the same skill in different contexts and increasing levels of challenge (Rousmaniere, 2016). Recent DP training manuals that use this strategy have been devised for the acquisition of skills from emotion-focused therapy (Goldman et al., 2021), motivational interviewing (Manuel et al., 2022), dialectical behavior therapy (Boritz et al., 2023), schema therapy (Behary et al., 2023), child and adolescent therapy (Bate et al., 2022), and more (Table 1.1).

Baker (2015, p. 383) delineated the training advantages of the simulation-based methods used in DP:

1. Training is conducted without patient involvement.
2. Mistakes can occur repeatedly without harm.
3. Performance can be recorded and assessed for future feedback.

Table 1.1 Comparing routine performance, conceptual learning, and deliberate practice

Activity	Definition	Examples
Routine performance	Performing work as usual	Providing psychotherapy
Conceptual learning	Learning activities without repeated rehearsal/practice and feedback	Attending lectures Reading clinical theory, models, and research
Procedural learning/deliberate practice	Repetitive rehearsal of specific skills with ongoing corrective feedback	Repeated behavioral roleplaying of a specific clinical skill (e.g., goal setting)

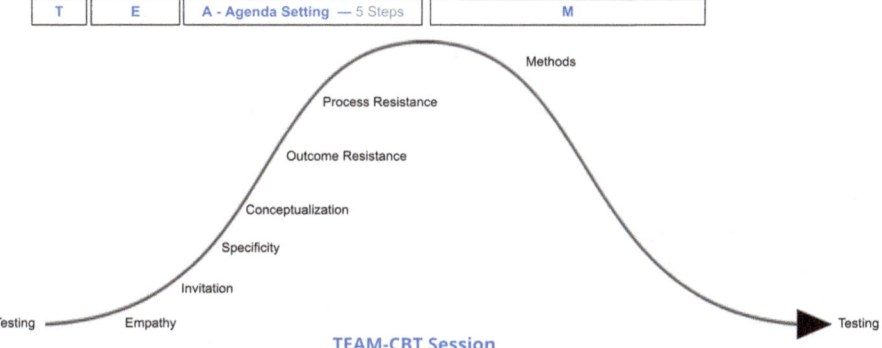

Fig. 1.2 The skills covered in this book

4. Procedures can be easily interrupted for feedback.
5. Exposure to difficulty and unusual scenarios can be created and rehearsed regularly.
6. Trainees can learn at their own rate.

There is growing consensus from prominent authors that DP methods might constitute an important advance in the future of mental health training and supervision (Miller et al., 2020; Wampold et al., 2019; Anderson & Perlman, 2020; Rousmaniere et al., 2017; Norcross & Karpiak, 2017). A recent number of studies provide preliminary support that DP methods reliably increase clinical skill acquisition (McLeod, 2021; Perlman et al., 2020; Westra et al., 2021; Di Bartolomeo et al., 2021; Anderson et al., 2020; Hill et al., 2020; Nikendei et al., 2019). It is our goal with this book to contribute to this exciting and growing literature on mental health training using DP methods. To do this, we have selected several TEAM CBT skills that we believe all mental health professionals should train routinely in order to achieve optimal clinical results (Fig. 1.2).

Illustration: TEAM-CBT Session Milestones and Flow
The session starts with the patient handing a brief mood survey to the therapist and is provided with immediate empathy and connection. The Invitation step kicks the work into gear, followed by a focus process with specificity. Conceptualization then leads to outcome Resistance work, followed by process Resistance work. By the time, we have reached methods, the heavy lifting is done and the Methods section rolls easily. Immediately after the session ends, the patient leaves behind another brief mood survey and therapy session evaluation

When we set out to write this book, we wanted to capture with simple exercises the essence and spirit of the TEAM-CBT approach and help you internalize it. Our goal is to make skills that are felt to be intangible, implicit, explicit, and trainable. Since TEAM-CBT is a process-oriented approach that offers a sequential series of steps for therapy, the skills we chose follow the steps and skills you would use sequentially in a therapy session.

This approach makes every encounter matter, even if it's brief. We have found that learning the TEAM-CBT skills set has helped our practice in every context, not only working with the higher functioning, affluent population of our Silicon Valley practice but also working with low-income, low-resource populations, such as in community mental health settings, or in the context of a single-session intervention, such as in the corrections system. And these skills have not only been applied to outpatients but also in brief high-acuity encounters in psychiatry hospital units, family sessions with social workers and case coordinators, as well as medication management meetings in a more medication-based practice or even a family medicine practice. Whatever the context of your work, whether you see patients with abundant time in a private practice setting week after week or only for 15-minute encounters, as well as everything in between, you will find these skills make every encounter more effective and helpful, relieving both you and your patients.

Follow the book sequentially, and you will be able to internalize the full map of the process of making therapy more effective with the TEAM-CBT approach. The first exercise, Testing (Skill 1), is made to help you feel more comfortable using measurement before, after, and throughout the session. The two Empathy exercises (2A and 2B) introduce you to a simple, powerful system for improving your therapeutic alliance and empathy skills. With the Invitation exercise (3), you will learn how to kick therapy into gear and then how to focus the work with Specificity (4). The Conceptualization step (5) is meant to help you know ahead of time what the likely Outcome and Process Resistance themes will be so you can help the patient bring them to conscious awareness and melt them away (6A and 6B, 7A and 7B). Once you have done all that, the Methods part (8–11) will be as easy as rolling down a hill. Assigning homework (12) is the last skill in the book. We use it here both to help you improve your homework assignment skill and to internalize the TEAM-CBT road map.

References

Anderson, T., & Perlman, M. R. (2020). Therapeutic interpersonal skills for facilitating the working alliance. In J. N. Fuertes (Ed.), *Working alliance skills for mental health professionals*. Oxford.

Anderson, T., Perlman, M. R., McCarrick, S. M., & McClintock, A. S. (2020). Modeling therapist responses with structured practice enhances facilitative interpersonal skills. *Journal of Clinical Psychology, 76*(4), 659–675.

Angelakis, I., Huggett, C., Gooding, P., Panagioti, M., & Hodkinson, A. (2022). Effectiveness of cognitive–behavioural therapies of varying complexity in reducing depression in adults: Systematic review and network meta-analysis. *The British Journal of Psychiatry*, 1–9.

Aviram, A., Westra, H. A., Constantino, M. J., & Antony, M. M. (2016). Responsive management of early resistance in cognitive–behavioral therapy for generalized anxiety disorder. *Journal of Consulting and Clinical Psychology, 84*(9), 783.

Baker, P. (2015). Preparedness and education in airway management. *Anesthesiology Clinics, 33*(2), 381–395.

Bate, J., Prout, T., Rousmaniere, T., & Vaz, A. (2022). *Deliberate practice in child and adolescent psychotherapy*. American Psychological Association.

Behary, W. T., Farrell, J. M., Vaz, A., & Rousmaniere, T. (2023). *Deliberate practice in schema therapy*. American Psychological Association.

Beidas, R. S., & Kendall, P. C. (2010). Training therapists in evidence-based practice: A critical review of studies from a systems-contextual perspective. *Clinical Psychology: Science and Practice, 17*(1), 1–30.

Beidas, R. S., Cross, W., & Dorsey, S. (2014). Show me, don't tell me: Behavioral rehearsal as a training and analogue fidelity tool. *Cognitive and Behavioral Practice, 21*(1), 1–11.

Burns, D., Westra, H., Trockel, M., & Fisher, A. (2013). Motivation and changes in depression. *Cognitive therapy and research, 37*, 368–379.

Boritz, T., McMain, S., Vaz, A., & Rousmaniere, T. (2023). *Deliberate practice in dialectical behavior therapy*. American Psychological Association.

Boswell, J. F., Farchione, T. J., Sauer-Zavala, S., Murray, H. W., Fortune, M. R., & Barlow, D. H. (2013). Anxiety sensitivity and interoceptive exposure: A transdiagnostic construct and change strategy. *Behavior Therapy, 44*(3), 417–431.

Boswell, J. F., Kraus, D. R., Miller, S. D., & Lambert, M. J. (2015). Implementing routine outcome monitoring in clinical practice: Benefits, challenges, and solutions. *Psychotherapy Research, 25*(1), 6–19.

Burns, D. D. (1980). *Feeling good, the new mood therapy*. Signet Books.

Burns, D. D. (1993). *Ten days to self-esteem: The leader's manual*. Quill/HarperCollins Publishers.

Burns, D. D. (1997). *Tools not schools for therapy*. Available as e-book on FeelingGood.com

Burns, D. D. (1999). *The feeling good handbook*. Plume.

Burns, D. D. (2010). *Feeling good together: The secret to making troubled relationships work*. Random House.

Carpenter, J. K., Andrews, L. A., Witcraft, S. M., Powers, M. B., Smits, J. A., & Hofmann, S. G. (2018). Cognitive behavioral therapy for anxiety and related disorders: A meta-analysis of randomized placebo-controlled trials. *Depression and Anxiety, 35*(6), 502–514.

Craske, M. G., Treanor, M., Conway, C. C., Zbozinek, T., & Vervliet, B. (2014). Maximizing exposure therapy: An inhibitory learning approach. *Behaviour Research and Therapy, 58*, 10–23.

Cross, W. F., Seaburn, D., Gibbs, D., Schmeelk-Cone, K., White, A. M., & Caine, E. D. (2011). Does practice make perfect? A randomized control trial of behavioral rehearsal on suicide prevention gatekeeper skills. *The Journal of Primary Prevention, 32*(3–4), 195.

Di Bartolomeo, A. A., Shukla, S., Westra, H. A., Shekarak Ghashghaei, N., & Olson, D. A. (2021). Rolling with resistance: A client language analysis of deliberate practice in continuing education for psychotherapists. *Counselling and Psychotherapy Research, 21*(2), 433–441.

Ericsson, K. A. (2003). Development of elite performance and deliberate practice: An update from the perspective of the expert performance approach. In J. L. Starkes & K. A. Ericsson (Eds.), *Expert performance in sports: Advances in research on sport expertise*. Human Kinetics.

Ericsson, K. A. (2004). Deliberate practice and the acquisition and maintenance of expert performance in medicine and related domains. *Academic Medicine, 79*(10), S70–S81.

Ericsson, K. A., & Pool, R. (2016). *Peak: Secrets from the new science of expertise*. Mifflin Harcourt.

Ericsson, K. A., Hoffman, R. R., Kozbelt, A., & Williams, A. M. (Eds.). (2018). *The Cambridge handbook of expertise and expert performance*. Cambridge University Press.

Fang, A., Sawyer, A. T., Asnaani, A., & Hofmann, S. G. (2013). Social mishap exposures for social anxiety disorder: An important treatment ingredient. *Cognitive and Behavioral Practice, 20*(2), 213–220.

Goldman, R. N., Vaz, A., & Rousmaniere, T. (2021). *Deliberate practice in emotion-focused therapy*. American Psychological Association.

Hayes, S. C., & Hofmann, S. G. (Eds.). (2018). *Process-based CBT: The science and core clinical competencies of cognitive behavioral therapy*. New Harbinger Publications.

Herschell, A. D., Kolko, D. J., Baumann, B. L., & Davis, A. C. (2010). The role of therapist training in the implementation of psychosocial treatments: A review and critique with recommendations. *Clinical Psychology Review, 30*(4), 448–466.

Hill, C. E., & Knox, S. (2013). Training and supervision in psychotherapy. In M. J. Lambert (Ed.), *Handbook of psychotherapy and behavior change* (6th ed., pp. 775–811). Wiley.

Hill, C. E., Kivlighan, D. M., III, Rousmaniere, T., Kivlighan, D. M., Jr., Gerstenblith, J. A., & Hillman, J. W. (2020). Deliberate practice for the skill of immediacy: A multiple case study of doctoral student therapists and clients. *Psychotherapy, 57*(4), 587.

Howick, J., Moscrop, A., Mebius, A., Fanshawe, T. R., Lewith, G., Bishop, F. L., et al. (2018). Effects of empathic and positive communication in healthcare consultations: A systematic review and meta-analysis. *Journal of the Royal Society of Medicine, 111*(7), 240–252.

Huppert, J. D., Kivity, Y., Barlow, D. H., Gorman, J. M., Shear, M. K., & Woods, S. W. (2014). Therapist effects and the outcome–alliance correlation in cognitive behavioral therapy for panic disorder with agoraphobia. *Behaviour Research and Therapy, 52*, 26–34.

Lambert, M. J., & Ogles, B. M. (1997). The effectiveness of psychotherapy supervision. In C. E. Watkins Jr. (Ed.), *Handbook of psychotherapy supervision* (pp. 421–446). Wiley.

Lambert, M. J., Whipple, J. L., & Kleinstäuber, M. (2018). Collecting and delivering progress feedback: A meta-analysis of routine outcome monitoring. *Psychotherapy, 55*(4), 520–537.

Lungu, A., Jun, J. J., Azarmanesh, O., Leykin, Y., & Chen, C. E. J. (2020). Blended care-cognitive behavioral therapy for depression and anxiety in real-world settings: Pragmatic retrospective study. *Journal of Medical Internet Research, 22*(7), e18723.

Manuel, J. K., Ernst, D., Rousmaniere, T., & Vaz, A. (2022). *Deliberate practice in motivational interviewing*. American Psychological Association.

McGaghie, W. C., Issenberg, S. B., Cohen, M. E. R., Barsuk, J. H., & Wayne, D. B. (2011). Does simulation-based medical education with deliberate practice yield better results than traditional clinical education? A meta-analytic comparative review of the evidence. *Academic Medicine: Journal of the Association of American Medical Colleges, 86*(6), 706.

McGaghie, W. C., Issenberg, S. B., Barsuk, J. H., & Wayne, D. B. (2014). A critical review of simulation-based mastery learning with translational outcomes. *Medical Education, 48*(4), 375–385.

McLeod, J. (2021). How students use deliberate practice during the first stage of counsellor training. *Counselling and Psychotherapy Research, 22*, 1–12.

Miller, S. D., Hubble, M. A., & Chow, D. (2020). *Better results: Using deliberate practice to improve therapeutic effectiveness*. American Psychological Association.

Nikendei, C., Huber, J., Ehrenthal, J. C., Herzog, W., Schauenburg, H., Schultz, J. H., & Dinger, U. (2019). Intervention training using peer role-play and standardised patients in psychodynamic psychotherapy trainees. *Counselling and Psychotherapy Research, 19*(4), 508–522.

Norcross, J. C., & Karpiak, C. P. (2017). Our best selves: Defining and actualizing expertise in psychotherapy. *The Counseling Psychologist, 45*(1), 66–75.

Perlman, M. R., Anderson, T., Foley, V. K., Mimnaugh, S., & Safran, J. D. (2020). The impact of alliance-focused and facilitative interpersonal relationship training on therapist skills: An RCT of brief training. *Psychotherapy Research, 30*(7), 871–884.

Persons, J. B., Koerner, K., Eidelman, P., Thomas, C., & Liu, H. (2016). Increasing psychotherapists' adoption and implementation of the evidence-based practice of progress monitoring. *Behaviour Research and Therapy, 76*, 24–31.

Pombo, S., Figueira, M. L., Walter, H., & Lesch, O. (2016). Motivational factors and negative affectivity as predictors of alcohol craving. *Psychiatry Research, 243*, 53–60.

Rousmaniere, T. (2016). *Deliberate practice for psychotherapists: A guide to improving clinical effectiveness.* Taylor & Francis.

Rousmaniere, T., Goodyear, R. K., Miller, S. D., & Wampold, B. E. (Eds.). (2017). *The cycle of excellence: Using deliberate practice to improve supervision and training.* Wiley.

Safran, J. D., & Muran, J. C. (2000). *Negotiating the therapeutic alliance: A relational treatment guide.* Guilford Press.

Solstad, S. M., Kleiven, G. S., Castonguay, L. G., & Moltu, C. (2021). Clinical dilemmas of routine outcome monitoring and clinical feedback: A qualitative study of patient experiences. *Psychotherapy Research, 31*(2), 200–210.

Vaz, A., & Rousmaniere, T. (2021). *Reaching for expertise: A primer on deliberate practice for psychotherapists.* Sentio Press.

Wampold, B. E., Lichtenberg, J. W., Goodyear, R. K., & Tracey, T. J. (2019). Clinical expertise. In S. Dimidjian (Ed.), *Evidence-based practice in action: Bridging clinical science and intervention* (pp. 152–166). Guilford Publications.

Westra, H. A., & Norouzian, N. (2018). Using motivational interviewing to manage process markers of ambivalence and resistance in cognitive behavioral therapy. *Cognitive Therapy and Research, 42*, 193–203.

Westra, H. A., Constantino, M. J., & Antony, M. M. (2016). Integrating motivational interviewing with cognitive-behavioral therapy for severe generalized anxiety disorder: An allegiance-controlled randomized clinical trial. *Journal of Consulting and Clinical Psychology, 84*(9), 768.

Westra, H. A., Norouzian, N., Poulin, L., Coyne, A., Constantino, M. J., Hara, K., et al. (2021). Testing a deliberate practice workshop for developing appropriate responsivity to resistance markers. *Psychotherapy, 58*(2), 175.

Zilcha-Mano, S., Muran, J. C., Hungr, C., Eubanks, C. F., Safran, J. D., & Winston, A. (2016). The relationship between alliance and outcome: Analysis of a two-person perspective on alliance and session outcome. *Journal of Consulting and Clinical Psychology, 84*(6), 484.

Part II
Deliberate Practice Exercises

Chapter 2
Instructions for the Deliberate Practice Exercises

Many training programs, trainers, and trainees will be unfamiliar with the deliberate practice (DP) methods used in this book. While most will have had experiences using some form of procedural training, such as clinical roleplays, DP exercises are different in some significant respects. Most notably, DP exercises encourage repetition and incremental refinement of the trainee's performance. This is achieved by designing exercises where clinical conversations do not veer into freeform roleplay or ongoing dialogue between the patient and the therapist, but instead focus on repeatedly providing the same stimulus so trainees may refine their use of a particular skill.

This chapter provides instructions that are common to all the exercises in this book. DP exercises in this book involve simulation-based role-plays of common clinical scenarios with patients. The DP role-play involves two to three people: one role-playing the therapist, another role-playing the patient, and whenever possible a trainer (professor/supervisor) observing and providing feedback. Every trainee will need their own copy of this book for practice purposes.

Another distinctive element of DP exercises is ongoing difficulty assessment and adjustments, so that practice targets each individual trainee's zone of proximal development. In essence, if an exercise is too easy for the trainee, it should be made harder; if too hard, it should be made easier; and if the exercise is providing a good challenge, then trainees should keep repeating the same simulation until it becomes too easy (see Step 4 in Table 2.1). The sections below provide more information on the steps necessary to ensure an effective practice session.

Structure of a Practice Session

We recommend a 60-minute time block for every exercise, structured as follows:

- **First 20 minutes:** Orientation. The trainer explains the skill and reads aloud the examples provided in each exercise.

© The Author(s), under exclusive license to Springer Nature Switzerland AG 2023   17
M. Katz et al., *Deliberate Practice of TEAM-CBT*, SpringerBriefs in Psychology,
https://doi.org/10.1007/978-3-031-46019-7_2

Table 2.1 Instruction for deliberate practice exercises

Step 1: The patient reads the first patient statement.
Step 2: The therapist improvises a response based on the exercise's skill criteria.
Step 3: The trainer (or, if not available, the person playing the patient) provides brief feedback on whether each skill criterion was met. Optionally, also check the example response provided at the end of the exercise.
Step 4: The patient repeats the same statement until it feels too easy for the therapist to meet the skill criteria. Proceed to the next patient statement **only when this is the case**.

For a demonstration of these steps in action, see: https://youtu.be/DhWf6rGMDL8

- **Middle 30 minutes:** Trainees perform the exercise in pairs. One trainee role-plays the therapist, another role-plays the patient. After 15 minutes of practice, trainees switch roles. If available, a trainer provides feedback on the therapist's interventions.
- **Final 10 minutes:** Debrief and final evaluation.

One trainer may teach multiple pairs of trainees at the same time by walking around the room and offering brief feedback to each pair.

How to Practice

The instructions table (Table 2.1) is common to all the exercises in this book, except Exercise #5, which follows a slightly revised format. Each step is mandatory, targeting a specific component of effective practice. Trainees and trainers should follow each step carefully and routinely revisit this table whenever necessary.

Below we provide more information on three elements of effective practice: The importance of skill criteria, the importance of feedback, and the debrief and final evaluation phase of practice.

Skill Criteria

Skill criteria are the observable verbal and nonverbal therapist behaviors that define the skill being practiced. Each of the first 12 exercises in this book provides skill criteria that make the skill being practiced more concrete and understandable. We have found that one common issue in most traditional training methods is the use of vague or broad language that does not lend itself well to effective skill building. For instance, many trainees would be understandably unsure if they were tasked with practicing "validation," with no further deconstruction of what this term means behaviorally. Hence, in this example, we deconstruct the skill of validation into observable skill criteria, such as the criterion: "Highlight what is reasonable, normal, or wise about the patient's response (e.g., thoughts, feelings, behaviors)."

Skill criteria are perhaps the single most important element of each DP exercise, in that they provide clear guidelines for what the trainee is attempting to do and clear observable behaviors trainers can evaluate trainees on and provide concrete feedback.

Feedback

Step 3 of the Instructions (Table 2.1) highlights the importance of providing ongoing feedback after each intervention attempted by the trainee playing the therapist. Feedback is an essential component of DP, providing the opportunity to give concrete, behavioral input that the trainees can take in and incrementally attempt to refine their interventions.

Most importantly, effective DP feedback includes the following two characteristics:

- **The trainer (or person playing patient) provides feedback focused on the exercise skill criteria and therapist's observable behaviors.** It is essential that feedback is not focused on discussing the patient statements, diagnoses, or broad mental health theory, but rather on the therapist's performance. Feedback should always link back to the skill criteria provided in each exercise. Trainers should evaluate if the trainee met each skill criterion, providing clear suggestions on how to refine the intervention if necessary. Trainers can also model an intervention that meets the exercise skill criteria, encouraging trainees to try again and refine their intervention.
- **Feedback should be brief.** We often find that trainees and trainers are understandably tempted to discuss theory and personal anecdotes when providing feedback. While this can be very interesting and gratifying, doing so will deter you from practicing skills. Instead, keep feedback specific, behavioral, and brief (1 minute maximum). Every person involved in the practice should encourage each other to quickly return to rehearsal and postpone longer theoretical discussions until after the practice has ended.

Debrief and Final Evaluation

Skill rehearsal proceeds for 30 minutes, with each trainee in the pair practicing as the therapist for 15 minutes. After 30 minutes of rehearsal, we reached the final phase of the practice session. In this phase, the participants debriefed on what was most challenging about practicing the skill and what they learned in the process. Importantly, trainers pinpoint specific individualized learning points for each trainee and encourage them to continue skill rehearsal by themselves or with a peer. Readings can also be assigned to complement skill rehearsal and answer theoretical questions that may have appeared during the practice.

Chapter 3
Testing: Using Measurement at the Start and End of Each Session

Skill Description

In TEAM-CBT, we ask patients to fill out a Brief Mood Survey right before and right after each session. At the end of each session, we also add an Evaluation of Therapy Session survey. We call this routine outcome measurement "Testing."

Before each session begins, the patient is asked to take inventory and report on different aspects of their mood using simple mood scales. This gives you, the therapist, a clear report in front of them of the patient's most current mood symptoms at the start of each session. You can then use the self-reported symptoms to connect with your patient about their feelings. This helps you have direct access to the heart of the matter and into an immediate, vulnerable tender discussion of your patient's most current feelings and emotions. It prevents the tendency of small talk or a less emotionally valent generic report from your patient about events in their lives of the previous week. Although it can sound technical and off-putting, using symptom measurement this way helps you get to work on meaningful emotional content more efficiently while saving precious session time.

As your patient leaves the session, they are asked to fill out a mood survey again, as well as evaluate the session itself for helpfulness, satisfaction, and warmth. Using these scales right before and after each session gives us two data points for each session and a way to connect to previous and following sessions. For those of us who have been practicing TEAM-CBT for a long time, it is no surprise to read the current data that show a near twofold increase in therapy effectiveness for therapists using routine outcome measurement (Lambert et al., 2018). It is also of little surprise that therapists find it difficult to implement routine outcome measurement, as we all often feel uncomfortable demanding certain things from our patients (Boswell et al., 2015).

When the therapist follows this protocol, each new session starts with a review of the patient's current feelings, while also comparing them to the previous session's

M. Katz et al., *Deliberate Practice of TEAM-CBT*, SpringerBriefs in Psychology, https://doi.org/10.1007/978-3-031-46019-7_3

report. This lets us assess progress, identify stuck points, and tend to the therapeutic relationship, while also connecting to the feelings in the here and now.

We also use measurement in many other moments of therapy. We ask patients to assess on a scale of 0–100% how strongly they feel different painful emotions they wish to get help with, or the degree of their belief in negative thoughts they identify. Later, after working on these feelings and thoughts, we cycle back and assess again to find out whether we are succeeding in improving their negative feelings and defeating their negative thoughts. In various ways, the concept of Testing in TEAM-CBT shows up repeatedly and is integrated into the therapy work.

Introducing routine "before" and "after" session surveys to the patient is typically done early in the therapeutic relationship, often during the very first encounter, intake session, or during a pre-first session call. Once introduced, following through and using it routinely becomes easier, though some degree of assertiveness on your part will be continuously required. For example, asking patients to take a moment to review the survey even when they have arrived late to the session without the survey requires a certain degree of assertiveness and gumption to follow through with. The following exercise is intended to help you feel more comfortable and prepared to introduce the system of testing to your patient.

Examples of This Skill in Practice

Example #1

Patient: I'm really looking forward to working with you!

Therapist: Me too! Let me quickly share with you how I like to keep track of your mood and how therapy is going for you. Before and after each session, you'll be asked to fill out a brief mood survey. (Criterion 1) This will take a few minutes of your time before and after we meet. (Criterion 4) Each session will start by quickly reviewing it so I can understand how you're feeling then and there. (Criterion 2) It will also serve as another way for us to track therapy progress. (Criterion 3) Can I show you the mood survey we'll use right now?

Example #2

Patient: I'm not sure how therapy works or what I will have to do.

Therapist: I am glad you asked that question. I work a little differently than other therapists. The first thing we are going to do at every session is have you fill in a brief check-in survey before and after every session. (Criterion 1) This is a critical part of our work (Criterion 4) because it will help us in two ways. The first is that it will help me to more fully understand how you are feeling so we are not missing anything important. (Criterion 2) The second is that it will help us to monitor the progress of our work together and make sure we are on the right track. (Criterion 3)

Example #3

Patient: Shall we start with me telling you all about my week?

Therapist: That is a great idea, but before we dive in I am going to have you fill out a brief mood survey that is a key tool we use in our work together. (Criterion 1) It will only take a couple minutes and I will have you fill it out again right after our session. (Criterion 4) It is kind of like an emotional and relationship thermometer that will assist me in more fully understanding how you are feeling (Criterion 2) and will also provide us a way to check our therapy progress to make sure we are on track. (Criterion 3)

Now it is your turn: Follow the Exercise Instructions and Skill Criteria (Table 3.1).

After 15 minutes of practice, the patient and therapist switch roles and start over.

For these next statements, the patient is pleasant and receptive.

Patient Statement #1 How does this therapy work? I have a lot of questions, but I am not sure where to start.

Patient Statement #2 I am really looking for the type of therapy where I know what is actually going on.

Patient Statement #3 I tried talk therapy, but I want something more tangible and productive.

Table 3.1 Criteria for "testing" exercise

The therapist improvises a response to each patient statement using the following criteria:
1. Redirect the conversation to introducing the use of surveys before and after each session.
2. Explain that it will help you better understand how the patient is feeling.
3. Explain that it will help both of you track progress and stuck points in therapy.
4. Convey that mood surveys before and after each session are expected.
Proceed to the next patient statement only when it is too easy for the therapist to meet all criteria.

Patient Statement #4 Where should I start?

> *For these next statements, the patient is somewhat receptive and somewhat open to getting to work.*

Patient Statement #5 My friend told me that it is important to tell my whole story, so I am ready.

Patient Statement #6 I feel heartbroken; my girlfriend just dumped me out of the blue.

Patient Statement #7 I really need to tell you more about my history; my mother is quite an unusual person.

Patient Statement #8 I really need to tell you about my dad. He did something really terrible this week; you won't believe it!

> *For these next statements, the patient is challenging and reluctant to get to work.*

Patient Statement #9 How do I know this therapy will be helpful? I've done therapy in the past, but it honestly didn't do me any good.

Patient Statement #10 There is something I need to tell you about what happened this week. I have been holding it in for two days and need to get it out right now.

Patient Statement #11 Are you one of those therapists who force people to fill out forms? I'm so sick of useless forms, can't we just get straight to the point?

Patient Statement #12 Listen, I know you were probably trained to ask me to write up forms. I don't blame you, that's what they told you to tell me. But c'mon, what's the point of another piece of paper?

Trainees should attempt to improvise their own responses before reading the example responses (Table 3.2).

Table 3.2 Example therapist responses: testing

	Patient statements	Example therapist responses
Patient Statement #1	How does this therapy work? I have a lot of questions but I am not sure where to start.	Excellent! Let me show you how it works. (Criterion 1) Right before and right after each session, I'll ask you to fill out a mood survey. (Criterion 4) This will help me understand better how you're feeling right as we start a session, (Criterion 2) track progress and bring stuck points to our attention. (Criterion 3)
Patient Statement #2	I am really looking for the type of therapy where I know what is actually going on.	Wonderful! I like that too. Let me explain how we will start and finish every session (Criterion 1). I will send you a mood survey that you will fill out (Criterion 4) that will help me understand you better (Criterion 2) and assist us in tracking how therapy is progressing. This is key to identifying what is working as well as what might be getting in the way, so we can customize our approach and be as effective as possible. (Criterion 3)
Patient Statement #3	I tried talk therapy, but I want something more tangible and productive.	Excellent! Let me introduce you to the way I like to use mood surveys. (Criterion 1) You'll be asked to fill them out right before and right after each session. (Criterion 4) This will help me understand better how you're feeling, (Criterion 2) help us track progress and stuck points in our work, and make sure we are being productive. (Criterion 3)
Patient Statement #4	Where should I start?	Great question. Let me share with you how we will start and end every session together using these testing forms. (Criterion 1) The mood forms that I require you to fill out help us in two ways. (Criterion 4) The first is that it helps me to get in tune with how you are feeling so I can more fully understand where you are at. (Criterion 2) The second is that it gives us important information about what is effective in our work and what might not be working. This is why we have you fill it out at the end of every session as well (Criterion 3).
Patient Statement #5	My friend told me that it is important to tell my whole story, so I am ready.	Absolutely. Let's first start by introducing you to how this kind of therapy works. (Criterion 4) We use mood surveys before and after each session. (Criterion 1) This will help me understand how you are feeling as we start each session (Criterion 2) as well as track progress and stuck points in therapy. (Criterion 3) Would you be willing to fill out a mood survey right now before we jump in?

(continued)

Table 3.2 (continued)

	Patient statements	Example therapist responses
Patient Statement #6	I feel heartbroken; my girlfriend just dumped me out of the blue.	That sounds painful. I would like to get a better understanding of how you are feeling, so before we go any further, I want you to fill out this mood survey. (Criterion 1) You will fill it out before and after every appointment so we can track our progress, uncover any stuck points, and make sure we are on the same page. (Criteria 2 and 3) Our research has shown that therapists are actually not that good at picking up on everything, so these mood surveys are an essential part of therapy to take away the guesswork. (Criterion 4)
Patient Statement #7	I really need to tell you more about my history; my mother is quite an unusual person.	Absolutely. I'm eager to hear and there's so much about you I'd like to learn more about! Before we start I'd like to introduce you to the use of surveys before and after each therapy session. (Criterion 1) This will help me understand better how you are feeling at the beginning and after each time we meet, (Criterion 2) track progress, and flush out stuck points in therapy. (Criterion 3) I use these surveys before and after sessions with all of my patients, is that something you'd be willing to do? (Criterion 4)
Patient Statement #8	I really need to tell you about my dad. He did something really terrible this week; you won't believe it!	That sounds important, and I am looking forward to hearing all about it. Before we jump into it, I am going to have you fill in this brief mood survey that is a critical component of our work together. (Criteria 1 and 4) I will have you complete it before and after every session to help me better understand how you are feeling. (Criterion 2) We will also use it to track our progress so we can identify what is working well in therapy and what might be barriers that are getting in the way of your goals. (Criterion 4)
Patient Statement #9	How do I know this therapy will be helpful? I've done therapy in the past, and it honestly didn't do me any good.	You've been disappointed in the past with therapy. I'm grateful you are here. One way we'll both know if it's helpful to you is by using mood surveys before and after each session. (Criterion 1) I do this with all of my patients. (Criterion 4) This will help us track progress and see whether therapy is working and identify stuck points. (Criterion 3) It will also help me better understand how you feel. (Criterion 2)
Patient Statement #10	There is something I need to tell you about what happened this week. I have been holding it in for two days and need to get it out right now.	Wow, that sounds important, and we will definitely take time to explore it. This may seem a little different but an important way for me to get the whole story and fully understand how you are feeling is to have you fill out this brief mood survey before we start. (Criteria 1 and 2) I will also have you fill it out (Criterion 4) after the session so we can check in on our progress and see if we are missing anything or if there is something we are doing that is working well. (Criterion 3)

(continued)

Table 3.2 (continued)

	Patient statements	Example therapist responses
Patient Statement #11	Are you one of those therapists who force people to fill out forms? I'm so sick of useless forms, can't we just get straight to the point?	Oh! I hear it's been completely useless for you! I do ask all of my patients to fill out mood surveys before and after each session. (Criterion 1) I don't know of any other way of providing effective therapy for you. I'm not sure if this is what you meant, but these mood surveys we use before and after each session are helpful to me to get an immediate report on how you are feeling right as we start (Criterion 2) and identify stuck points in therapy. (Criterion 3) But I recognize it's not everyone's cup of tea and it may mean you won't want to work with me. (Criterion 4)
Patient Statement #12	Listen, I know you were probably trained to ask me to write up forms. I don't blame you, that's what they told you to tell me. But c'mon, what's the point of another piece of paper?	That is such a good question, and one I have asked myself. I use forms a little differently than others and I am happy to explain my approach. (Criterion 1) First is that I don't actually ask people to fill them out, and this may sound harsh, but I have a requirement that the brief mood surveys are filled out before and after every session. You see, I don't know how to work with people without them. It is a bit like asking a car mechanic to fix your car without using his tools, these are two of my main tools. (Criterion 4) The second is that I use them primarily to hear and understand you better. Our research has revealed that, sadly, therapists are not very good at guessing how people are feeling so these forms bring that to life for us. (Criterion 2) They also provide essential tracking information so we can identify what is and what is not working in therapy so we can adjust with accuracy. (Criterion 3)

References

Boswell, J. F., Kraus, D. R., Miller, S. D., & Lambert, M. J. (2015). Implementing routine outcome monitoring in clinical practice: Benefits, challenges, and solutions. *Psychotherapy Research, 25*(1), 6–19.

Lambert, M. J., Whipple, J. L., & Kleinstäuber, M. (2018). Collecting and delivering progress feedback: A meta-analysis of routine outcome monitoring. *Psychotherapy, 55*(4), 520–537.

Chapter 4
Empathy Training Part 1: Disarming, Thought Empathy, and Feeling Empathy Techniques

Introduction

The **E** in TEAM-CBT stands for Empathy. It is essential for the success of therapy that patients find their therapists to be warm, supportive, understanding, and on the same wavelength. We view great empathy as a necessary but insufficient part of the skill set of an effective therapist. We assume all therapists have flawed empathy skills that need to be endlessly practiced and continuously improved. Accepting that you are not very good at empathy is hard. The good news is that it offers an opportunity to improve. TEAM-CBT therapists spend a lot of time learning these empathy skills and, in turn, teach those same skills to patients to help them improve their communication and relationships in their own lives.

In TEAM-CBT, empathy can be distilled into five basic skills (with the second one split into two components), called 'Five Secrets',[1] for short:

The Five Secrets For Effective Communication are as follows:

1. **Disarming**: Find a grain of truth in what the patient is saying and agree with it wholeheartedly.
2. **Thought and Feel Empathy**: Repeat verbatim a part of what the patient said. Name some of the feelings they are conveying (especially anger).
3. **I Feel Statements**: Openly name some of the emotions that you, the therapist, are feeling at the moment.
4. **Stroking/Affirmation:** Find something you genuinely like and admire about the patient and share it with them.
5. **Inquiry**: Ask questions that lead the patient to share more with you.

---

[1] Dr. Burns coined the term Five Secrets for Effective Communication, even though there are actually six. Secret #2: Thought and Feel Empathy is divided into two very different techniques: Thought Empathy and Feeling Empathy. We will practice all of them in this chapter.

M. Katz et al., *Deliberate Practice of TEAM-CBT*, SpringerBriefs in Psychology, https://doi.org/10.1007/978-3-031-46019-7_4

Mastering these five straightforward techniques is all that you need to become a master communicator and empathic listener. However, these techniques can be surprisingly counterintuitive and anxiety provoking to use in the heat of the moment.

Unlike the sequential steps of Agenda Setting, designed to melt away resistance to change, which you will practice later in the book (Exercises 3–7). The Five Secrets of Effective Communication are not delivered in any specific order or formula. Additionally, you do not need to use all of the techniques every time you speak. In fact, if you do so, you will likely be too verbose and not allow your patient enough space to talk.

Skill Description

In this exercise, we will practice three of the Five Secrets for Effective Communication techniques: Disarming, Thought Empathy, and Feeling Empathy:

1. **The Disarming Technique** can be seen as the polar opposite of being defensive. When a patient says something, we do not agree with, we have an overwhelming urge to explain or try to show them our point of view. This inevitably leads to the patient feeling less understood, on the opposite team of us, and digging their heels in. The Disarming Technique helps us respond with agreement. The more outrageous or unkind the patient statement seems to us, the more challenging it will be to find truth in it, agree with it wholeheartedly, and put our patient at ease.

   Disarming is relevant in many different patient contexts, including ruptures and other challenging moments. The key to the success of this technique is to wholeheartedly agree, and not qualify it, even if you only agree with a small grain of truth in the patient's words. The patient statements in this exercise will cover different common challenges to help you prepare for such moments.

2. **Thought Empathy** is straightforward. Repeat the verbatim part of what the patient said, without any changes, additions, or interpretations, and without adding anything in your own words. We often feel anxious using Thought Empathy for fear of sounding silly to our patient's ears, like parroting. When we overcome this anxiety and use Thought Empathy more, our patients feel better understood and listened to.

3. **Feeling Empathy:** Name some of the feelings you are sensing your patient is experiencing such as Sad, Down, Disappointed, Angry, Annoyed, Excited, Worried, Tense, Afraid, Anxious, etc. Sometimes, the patient will actually name their feelings and you will only need to repeat them. Often, however, you will need to guess. We can feel afraid of guessing wrong, sounding presumptive, or disconnected from the patient. As a result, we avoid naming the patient's feelings. This technique asks you to overcome that fear and name feelings you sense your patient is displaying, even if you might get it wrong.

Examples of This Skill in Practice

Example #1
Patient: I'm so tired of being depressed.

Therapist: You are absolutely right, being depressed is so deeply tiring! (Criteria 1 and 2) I imagine you might be feeling overwhelmed, discouraged, and frustrated as well (Criterion 3)

Example #2
Patient: I'm so stressed and anxious with all the pressure at work.

Therapist: The pressure at work has been too much! (Criteria 1 and 2) No wonder you've been so stressed out and anxious. (Criteria 1 and 3)

Example #3
Patient: I thought you said you could help me, but we are not getting anywhere and this therapy is costing a fortune.

Therapist: You're absolutely right; I haven't been as helpful to you as I had hoped and I haven't been valuable enough for you to justify how much it's costing you. (Criteria 1 and 2) You have every right to feel disappointed and annoyed with me for that. (Criterion 3)

> **Now it is your turn: Follow the Exercise Instructions and Skill Criteria (Table 4.1).**

> **After 15 minutes of practice, the patient and therapist switch roles and start over.**

> *For these next statements, the patient is pleasant and receptive.*

Patient Statement #1 Last week, I had such an awful panic attack, and then again two days later, now I feel super fragile and shaken up.

Table 4.1 Criteria for empathy training Part 1 exercise

The therapist improvises a response to each patient statement using the following criteria:
1. Find the truth in what the patient is saying and completely agree with it. (Disarming Technique)
2. Repeat verbatim part of what the patient said. (Thought Empathy)
3. Name emotions the patient stated or emotions they may be feeling. (Feeling Empathy)
Proceed to the next patient statement only when it is too easy for the therapist to meet all criteria.

Patient Statement #2 I just can't seem to get a handle on my procrastinating. It is so frustrating to be stuck like this.

Patient Statement #3 I can't seem to go to bed on time, then wake up in the afternoon and feel crappy for the rest of the day.

Patient Statement #4 Starting college has been so hard because none of my friends came with me, and I feel so alone.

For these next statements, the patient is somewhat receptive and somewhat open to getting to work.

Patient Statement #5 Whenever I meet a new person at work, I feel so anxious that I almost have a panic attack.

Patient Statement #6 My mind is racing all the time and I think I am losing it. It's overwhelming and just seems to be getting worse.

Patient Statement #7 I sometimes think we shouldn't have had another child, and that makes me feel like a monster.

Patient Statement #8 I really messed up and now I only see my kids half the time. I worry constantly when they are with my ex.

For these next statements, the patient is challenging and reluctant to get to work.

Patient Statement #9 I want to quit, but right now the only thing I can think of that helps me is smoking weed.

Patient Statement #10 I think there's a problem with me; I'm always feeling angry.

Patient Statement #11 My boss is an asshole; they treat me like shit, and I hate my job.

Patient Statement #12 I think we have a special bond. You are such a good listener. Maybe we could get together for coffee sometime so I can get to know you better.

Trainees should attempt to improvise their own responses before reading the example responses (Table 4.2).

Table 4.2 Example therapist responses: empathy Part 1

	Patient statements	Example therapist responses
Patient Statement #1	Last week I had such an awful panic attack, and then again two days later, now I feel super fragile and shaken up	That makes complete sense that you would feel super fragile and shaken up after having an awful panic attack and then another one two days later. (Criteria 1 and 2) I imagine that you might be feeling stressed, anxious, and overwhelmed. (Criterion 3)
Patient Statement #2	I just can't get a handle on my procrastinating. It is so frustrating to be stuck like this.	You haven't made the progress you've been wishing for in overcoming procrastination. (Criterion 1) It makes complete sense that you're feeling so frustrated and stuck. (Criteria 1–3)
Patient Statement #3	I can't seem to go to bed on time, then wake up in the afternoon and feel crappy for the rest of the day	That has to be frustrating and exhausting, (Criterion 3) not being able to go to bed on time, waking up in the afternoon, and feeling crappy for the rest of the day. (Criteria 1 and 2)
Patient Statement #4	Starting college has been so hard because none of my friends came with me, and I feel so alone.	You feel so alone. (Criteria 2 and 3) Starting college has been so hard without your friends. (Criteria 1 and 2)
Patient Statement #5	Whenever I meet a new person at work I feel so anxious, I almost have a panic attack.	Meeting new people at work is stressful. (Criterion 1) It sounds like it makes you feel so anxious that you almost have a panic attack. That has to be terrifying when it happens. (Criteria 1–3)
Patient Statement #6	My mind is racing all the time and I think I am losing it. It's overwhelming and just seems to be getting worse.	You're just feeling worse and worse. (Criterion 1) Your mind is racing all the time, (Criterion 2) and you feel completely overwhelmed. (Criterion 3)
Patient Statement #7	I sometimes think we shouldn't have had another child, and that makes me feel like a monster.	You really care about your children, so it makes sense that you are feeling guilty and ashamed when you think that you shouldn't have had another child. (Criteria 1–3) It even makes you feel like a monster, which must be painful. (Criteria 2 and 3)
Patient Statement #8	I really messed up and now I only see my kids half the time. I worry constantly when they are with my ex.	You're feeling responsible for seeing your kids only half the time (Criteria 1 and 2) and are now constantly worried (Criterion 3) when they are with your ex. (Criterion 2)
Patient Statement #9	I want to quit, but right now the only thing I can think of that helps me is smoking weed.	Smoking weed is the one thing that has helped you so it makes sense that it is the only thing you can think of right now. (Criteria 1, 2) That has to be frustrating and discouraging when you want to quit but don't have anything else right now. (Criterion 3)
Patient Statement #10	I thought you said you could help me but we are not getting anywhere and this therapy is costing a fortune.	Absolutely, (Criterion 1) this therapy is costing you a fortune, and it hasn't really gotten you anywhere. (Criteria 1 and 2) You're probably feeling annoyed with me and disappointed. (Criterion 3)
Patient Statement #11	My boss is an asshole; they treat me like crap, and I hate my job.	I would hate my job too if they treated me like crap and my boss was an asshole. (Criteria 1 and 2) You must be feeling stuck, frustrated, and angry and justifiably so. (Criterion 3)

(continued)

Table 4.2 (continued)

	Patient statements	Example therapist responses
Patient Statement #12	I think we have a special bond. You are such a good listener. Maybe we could get together for coffee sometime, so I can get to know you better.	It is absolutely a special bond, (Criteria 1 and 2) and one with safety boundaries that I would never betray you by breaking. I respect you tremendously and would never betray the trust you placed in me by meeting socially. I imagine this may feel rejecting to hear. (Criterion 3) What's it like for you hearing me say that right now?

Chapter 5
Empathy Training Part 2: Stroking, "I Feel" Statements, and Inquiry Techniques

Skill Description

In this exercise, we will practice the rest of the Five Secrets for Effective Communication: Stroking, I Feel Statements, and Inquiry.

1. **Stroking/Affirmation**: This skill asks you to specifically name something you **genuinely** like and admire about your patient. You are doing it with the purpose of making them feel at ease, safe, and liked. Your opinion of them is important to your patients. Hearing that you genuinely like something about them will help them feel more comfortable. But it can feel awkward for you to give compliments to patients. You may worry that they will think you are being inappropriate or disingenuous. You will need to overcome these fears in order to use this technique. Sometimes it can be hard to find something you like and admire. It could be implicit, and you may need to pause to think about what good qualities you see in your patient.

2. **I Feel Statements:** This may be the hardest of the Five Secrets for Effective Communication. We are asked to name some of our own feelings as therapists, including negative ones. We always name our feelings with the intention of helping our patients. Without I Feel Statements, the therapeutic relationship can feel stiff and clinical. You may balk at this skill first and worry that the patient will see you as inappropriate and self-absorbed.

3. **Inquiry:** Ask gentle questions that invite the patient to talk. It is not always in the form of a question. It could be a request, such as "Tell me more" or "I'd like to hear more about that." It often acts in conversation as a way to pass the button for talking to the patient. If you sense you are talking too much as a therapist, go to inquiry.

© The Author(s), under exclusive license to Springer Nature Switzerland AG 2023   35
M. Katz et al., *Deliberate Practice of TEAM-CBT*, SpringerBriefs in Psychology,
https://doi.org/10.1007/978-3-031-46019-7_5

Examples of This Skill in Practice

Context: Imagine these patient statements are stated by a somewhat challenging patient you have been working with for a few sessions.

Example #1
Patient: I'm so tired of being depressed.
Therapist: You really want more from life and I appreciate your commitment to working to get there. (Criterion 1) I feel a little sad to hear that you have been feeling so tired and depressed. (Criterion 2) Tell me more about what it is like for you? (Criterion 3)

Example #2
Patient: I'm so stressed and anxious with all the pressure at work.
Therapist: You have such a high work ethic. (Criterion 1) I feel sad thinking about how stressed you've been feeling and kind of annoyed with your workplace putting so much pressure on you. (Criterion 2) Can you tell me more? (Criterion 3)

Example #3
Patient: I think there's a problem with me, I'm always feeling angry.
Therapist: I love your integrity, (Criterion 1) and my heart feels a little sore (Criterion 2) thinking about how crappy you've been feeling about yourself. Can you share more with me about how you're feeling? (Criterion 3)

> **Now it is your turn: Follow the Exercise Instructions and Skill Criteria (Table 5.1).**

> **After 15 minutes of practice, the patient and therapist switch roles and start over.**

Table 5.1 Criteria for empathy training Part 2 exercise

The therapist improvises a response to each patient statement using the following criteria:
1. State something you genuinely like and admire about your patient. (Stroking/Affirmation)
2. Name some of the feelings you are currently experiencing at the moment. (I Feel Statements)
3. Ask open-ended questions inviting the patient to share more. (Inquiry)
Proceed to the next patient statement <u>only</u> when it is too easy for the therapist to meet all criteria.

Context: Imagine these patient statements are stated by a patient you have been working with for a few sessions.

For these next statements, the patient is pleasant and receptive.

Patient Statement #1 Last week, I had such an awful panic attack, and then again two days later, now I feel super fragile and shaken up.

Patient Statement #2 I just can't seem to get a handle on my procrastinating. It is so frustrating to be stuck like this.

Patient Statement #3 I can't seem to go to bed on time, then wake up in the afternoon and feel crappy for the rest of the day.

Patient Statement #4 Starting college has been so hard because none of my friends came with me and I feel so alone.

For these next statements, the patient is somewhat receptive and somewhat open to getting to work.

Patient Statement #5 Whenever I meet a new person at work, I feel so anxious that I almost have a panic attack.

Patient Statement #6 My mind is racing all the time, and I think I am losing it. It's overwhelming and just seems to be getting worse.

Patient Statement #7 I sometimes think we shouldn't have had another child, and that makes me feel like a monster.

Patient Statement #8 I really messed up, and now I only see my kids half the time. I worry constantly when they are with my ex. I just care about them so much.

For these next statements, the patient is challenging and reluctant to get to work.

Patient Statement #9 Right now, the only thing I can think of that helps me is smoking weed.

Patient Statement #10 I thought you said you could help me, but we are not getting anywhere, and this therapy is costing a fortune.

Patient Statement #11 My boss is an asshole; they treat me like shit, and I hate my job.

Patient Statement #12 I think we have a special bond. You are such a good listener. Maybe we could get together for coffee sometime, so I can get to know you better.

Trainees should attempt to improvise their own responses before reading the example responses (Table 5.2).

Table 5.2 Example therapist responses: empathy Part 2

	Patient statements	Example therapist responses
Patient Statement #1	Last week, I had such an awful panic attack, and then again two days later, now I feel super fragile and shaken up	It is apparent that you are very determined to get a handle on this anxiety. (Criterion 1) I feel a bit sad to hear how intense it has been for you. (Criterion 2) Tell me more about what that is like for you? (Criterion 3)
Patient Statement #2	I just can't get a handle on my procrastinating. It is so frustrating to be stuck like this.	I see and admire how important it is to you to overcome procrastination and that you hold yourself to high standards. (Criterion 1) I feel sad (Criterion 2) hearing how stuck you feel. Can you share more with me? (Criterion 3)
Patient Statement #3	I can't seem to go to bed on time, then wake up in the afternoon and feel crappy for the rest of the day	I admire your determination in searching for a way to get out of this rut with your sleeping pattern. (Criterion 1) I feel crappy too when my sleep is off track. At the same time, I am excited about the potential of working together on this. (Criterion 2) Help me get a better sense of how you are feeling about it. (Criterion 3)
Patient Statement #4	Starting college has been so hard because none of my friends came with me and I feel so alone.	Your friends are so important to you. (Criterion 1) I feel sad (Criterion 2) thinking of you all alone through the hardships of starting college. Can you tell me more about how you've been feeling? (Criterion 3)
Patient Statement #5	Whenever I meet a new person at work, I feel so anxious that I almost have a panic attack.	It seems like doing well at work and making a good impression with new people is important to you. (Criterion 1) I feel honored that you would invite me into your journey as it sounds painful and terrifying. (Criterion 2) Tell me a bit more about how it feels in those situations. (Criterion 3)

(continued)

Table 5.2 (continued)

	Patient statements	Example therapist responses
Patient Statement #6	My mind is racing all the time and I think I am losing it. It's overwhelming and just seems to be getting worse.	I can see how important it is to you to be on top of things and not lose it. (Criterion 1) I feel a little overwhelmed just hearing how much you're going through. (Criterion 2) Can you tell me more? (Criterion 3)
Patient Statement #7	I sometimes think we shouldn't have had another child, and that makes me feel like a monster.	It is clear that being a loving and caring parent is a high value of yours. (Criterion 1) I feel a little sad to hear that you are struggling with the challenges that having another child has brought. (Criterion 2) I would love to hear more about what that is like for you? (Criterion 3)
Patient Statement #8	I really messed up, and now I only see my kids half the time. I worry constantly when they are with my ex.	Your kids mean everything to you; you are such a caring parent. (Criterion 1) I feel sad thinking about you beating yourself up like this and feeling so guilty as well as worried for your kids. (Criterion 2) Can you tell me more about what it's been like for you? (Criterion 3)
Patient Statement #9	Right now, the only thing I can think of that helps me is smoking weed.	Full respect to you for searching out options to get relief. (Criterion 1) I am grateful that you reached out to me for some support. At the same time, I am feeling concerned to hear how stuck you have been and the only solution you can think of is smoking weed. (Criterion 2) Perhaps you can help me understand how hard this has been for you. (Criterion 3)
Patient Statement #10	I thought you said you could help me, but we are not getting anywhere, and this therapy is costing a fortune.	You have every right to feel annoyed and disappointed. You've been doing your part, faithfully showing up to therapy and doing the work. (Criterion 1) I feel bad that I've disappointed you and haven't delivered the results you've been longing for. (Criterion 2) I care about you and want you to get better. Can you share more with me? (Criterion 3)
Patient Statement #11	My boss is an asshole; they treat me like crap, and I hate my job.	You deserve to be treated with respect and you know what that is supposed to be like at work. (Criterion 1) It is disappointing to hear that your boss treats you poorly and you hate your job. (Criterion 2) That has to be so difficult. How does it feel to be in that situation every day? (Criterion 3)
Patient Statement #12	I think we have a special bond. You are such a good listener. Maybe we could get together for coffee sometime, so I can get to know you better.	You are a very kind and loving person, and I genuinely care about you. (Criterion 1) I feel bad, (Criterion 2) as I may have given you the wrong message. I see our therapy relationship as sacred and safe and I never meet with my patients socially. What's it like for you hearing me say that right now? (Criterion 3)

(continued)

Chapter 6
Changing Gears: Invitation

Skill Description

The five steps of Agenda Setting are a sequential set of techniques in TEAM-CBT aimed at melting away resistance to change. They take place after a safe bond has been established with the patient and before cognitive and behavioral techniques are employed to overcome the specific challenges at hand. The five steps are as follows:

1. Invitation
2. Specificity
3. Conceptualization
4. Outcome Resistance
5. Process Resistance

The first two steps, Invitation and Specificity, focus the work on a particular problem and point in time. Step 3, Conceptualization, focuses further and helps predict why the patient may not want to change or do the work required for change. Step 4, Outcome Resistance, helps the patient work through the good and great reasons *not* to change. The final step, Process Resistance, confronts the patient with the work needed in order to bring about the change they decided on.

The first step, Invitation, aims to shift from general talking and listening toward a focus on a specific problem the patient is seeking help with. Taking this seemingly straightforward step often brings up anxiety for therapists in the therapy room, as it requires significant assertiveness and may feel like an interruption of the patient's flow of natural conversation. Failure to use this technique results in therapy that may be supportive but meandering and that underuses the full scope of therapeutic techniques a CBT therapist has to offer. A good Invitation step is one that is done earlier in the therapy hour; summarizes the patient's challenges; offers to "roll up our sleeves" and focus on one challenge; conveys hope, warmth, and care; and ends with the option for the patient to continue talking, which is termed "open hands."

M. Katz et al., *Deliberate Practice of TEAM-CBT*, SpringerBriefs in Psychology,
https://doi.org/10.1007/978-3-031-46019-7_6

Examples of This Skill in Practice

Context: All patient statements occur early in the session.

Example #1
Patient: (depressive and anxious): I'm struggling today. I feel very down and depressed. I write out to-do lists but never get around to them; my dad is pressuring me all the time, and I'm super stressed about paying off my car loan.

Therapist: You've mentioned problems with depression, anxiety, procrastination, and relationships, and I can see how painful they have been for you. (Criterion 1) I'm wondering if you'd like some help with any one of them today (Criterion 2) or if you need more time to just talk and have me listen. (Criterion 3)

Example #2
Patient: (anxious and depressed): I just can't seem to overcome this anxiety, and I feel like such a failure all the time. I really need to figure this out.

Therapist: My heart goes out to you. You've been suffering so much with anxiety and sadness and feeling like a failure (Criterion 1). I'm wondering if you'd like some help with one of these problems today, and whether now would be a good time to get started, (Criterion 2) or perhaps you need more time to just talk and have me listen? What would you prefer? (Criterion 3)

Example #3
Patient: (sad): I'm struggling today; I'm in a bad spot with my girlfriend.

Therapist: Being in a bad spot in your relationship is a struggle. (Criterion 1) Is now a good time for us to roll up our sleeves and get to work on your relationship (Criterion 2), or would you like a little more time to tell me what that has been like for you? (Criterion 3)

> **Now it is your turn: Follow the Exercise Instructions and Skill Criteria (Table 6.1).**

> **After 15 minutes of practice, the patient and therapist switch roles and start over.**

Table 6.1 Criteria for invitation practice exercise

The therapist improvises a response to each patient statement using the following criteria:
1. Provide a brief empathetic summary of the patient's problems.
2. Explicitly invite the patient to get to work on the problem of the patient's choice.
3. Provide the option of continuing talking (open hands).
Proceed to the next patient statement only when it is too easy for the therapist to meet all criteria.

Context: All patient statements below occur early in the session.

Patient Statement #1 I have been struggling with feelings of depression and sadness and need some help with it.

Patient Statement #2 I need to figure out a way to beat this anxiety, and I will do whatever it takes.

Patient Statement #3 I really need to have someone show me how to get out of this rut of procrastination.

Patient Statement #4 There are two things bothering me: the first is feeling so depressed and the second is that it stresses me out that I can't seem to beat it.

Patient Statement #5 I am always stressed, no one really understands how hard it is, and everyone just wants to tell me what to do.

Patient Statement #6 I feel so worthless and just don't know how to feel better. My parents are always pressuring me and I have no motivation.

Patient Statement #7 I really need help with feeling depressed, my relationship is falling apart, I drink too much and I am super anxious about the new job starting next week.

Patient Statement #8 There are two main things bothering me. The first is the breakdown with my sister and the second is feeling lonely and wanting to be in a committed relationship.

Patient Statement #9 I want help getting over this depression, and my relationship is a mess too. But everyone expects me to do all the work.

Patient Statement #10 I feel so hopeless and just don't know how to feel better. My boss is always criticizing me, and I have no motivation.

Patient Statement #11 I have tried everything and nothing ever works to feel better.

Patient Statement #12 I don't know what I need today. Between the annoying way my sister is acting, the house renovation, the credit card payments, the panic attacks, the frustration with my kids' school schedule, and this depression, I am not sure where to even start.

Trainees should attempt to improvise their own responses before reading the example responses (Table 6.2)

Table 6.2 Example therapist responses: invitation

	Patient statements	Example therapist responses
Patient Statement #1	I have been struggling with feelings of depression and sadness and need some help with it.	You've been struggling with so much depression and sadness. (Criterion 1) Is now a good time for us to roll up our sleeves and get to work to help you with these feelings, (Criterion 2) or would you rather just share with me more about them and about what has been going on for you? (Criterion 3)
Patient Statement #2	I need to figure out a way to beat this anxiety, and I will do whatever it takes.	I love helping people overcome anxiety. (Criterion 1) Is now a good time to start and get to work on overcoming your anxiety, (Criterion 2) or would you like to share more about what it has been like for you first? (Criterion 3)
Patient Statement #3	I really need to have someone show me how to get out of this rut of procrastination.	I'd love to help you overcome the rut of procrastination. (Criterion 1) Is this something you'd like for us to work and focus on right now, (Criterion 2) or would you rather just share with me more about what it has been like for you? (Criterion 3)
Patient Statement #4	There are two things bothering me: the first is feeling so depressed and the second is that it stresses me out that I can't seem to beat it.	Would now be a good time to roll up our sleeves (Criterion 2) and focus on either of these feelings of depression or on the stress of not being able to beat it? (Criterion 1) Or would you like to first share with me some more about what has been going on for you? (Criterion 3)
Patient Statement #5	I am always stressed, no one really understands how hard it is, and everyone just wants to tell me what to do.	How painful it is to always feel stressed and not be understood. How annoying it is that everyone is always trying to fix you! (Criterion 1) Would now be a good time to roll up our sleeves and work on one of these problems, (Criterion 2) or perhaps it would be better for me to just continue to only provide you with a listening ear, warmth, and support? (Criterion 3)
Patient Statement #6	I feel so worthless and just don't know how to feel better. My parents are always pressuring me and I have no motivation.	You've shared how unmotivated and worthless and stuck you're feeling, not knowing how to feel better and how much pressure you feel from your parents. (Criterion 1) Would now be a good time to roll up our sleeves and get to work on one of these issues (Criterion 2), or would you prefer to just continue to share with me about what it has been like for you? (Criterion 3)

(continued)

Table 6.2 (continued)

	Patient statements	Example therapist responses
Patient Statement #7	I really need help with feeling depressed, my relationship is falling apart, I drink too much and I am super anxious about the new job starting next week.	There's so much going on! (Criterion 1) Would now be a good time to roll up our sleeves and get to work on one of the problems you've mentioned? (Criterion 2) Depression, relationship difficulties, anxiety, or drinking too much? Or would you rather just continue to share with me more about what it's been like for you and only receive warmth and support? (Criterion 3)
Patient Statement #8	There are two main things bothering me. The first is the breakdown with my sister and the second is feeling lonely and wanting to be in a committed relationship.	Would now be a good time to roll up our sleeves and get to work (Criterion 2) on either the breakdown with your sister or wanting to be in a relationship (Criterion 1), or would you rather share with me more about these issues or other issues first? (Criterion 3)
Patient Statement #9	I want help getting over this depression, and my relationship is a mess too. But everyone expects me to do all the work.	Everyone expects you to work work work (Criterion 1). Would now be a good time to focus on this issue and help you with it, or any of the other issues you've mentioned like depression and relationship challenges, (Criterion 2) or is this one of those times you really only want to share and be listened to (Criterion 3)?
Patient Statement #10	I feel so hopeless and just don't know how to feel better. My boss is always criticizing me, and I have no motivation.	Would now be a good time to get to work and help you (Criterion 2) either with the feelings of hopelessness, not knowing how to feel better, or the challenges with your boss, (Criterion 1) or would you rather work on something else or maybe just be listened to? (Criterion 3)
Patient Statement #11	I have tried everything and nothing ever works to feel better.	It must be so frustrating when you have tried everything and nothing has worked. (Criterion 1) If you would like more time to tell me about what this is like for you that would be important and I am fully in support if that is what you want. (Criterion 3) I would also be on board with you if you want to explore getting to work and investigating a different way to tackle this depression. (Criterion 2) I am not sure what the answer is, but I do have some powerful tools and would love to journey with you to discover the relief you are seeking. (Criterion 1)

(continued)

Table 6.2 (continued)

	Patient statements	Example therapist responses
Patient Statement #12	I don't know what I need today. Between the annoying way my sister is acting, the house renovation, the credit card payments, the panic attacks, the frustration with my kids' school schedule, and this depression, I am not sure where to even start.	It sounds like you are not sure what you need today. (Criterion 1) You listed a number of areas including the annoying way your sister is acting, the house renovation, the credit card payments, the panic attacks, the frustration with your kids' school schedule, and the depression. (Criterion 1) On the one hand, I would love to offer you more than listening and support. (Criterion 2) At the same time, I am not hearing that you are asking for that right now. (Criterion 3) Would now be a good time to get to work, or did you want to share more of the details? (Criterion 3)

Chapter 7
Getting Focused: Specificity

Skill Description

Specificity is the second step in agenda setting, which is done following a clearly accepted invitation by the patient to begin work (Chap. 6).

In order to help patients with their depression, anxiety, addiction, relationship problems, or anything else, we must pinpoint a moment in time when they were experiencing their difficulty. Once the therapist discovers the skills, methods, and solutions that work in helping them with this one moment in time, those same methods will likely work for other times when the patient is struggling with the same type of problem.

For this exercise, the therapist should start each response by wholeheartedly agreeing with the patients' choice of problem to work on. This is important because it ensures that we agree and follow the patient's agenda rather than pushing our own.

After this, the therapist's role is to gently guide the patient to think about a moment in time when they were struggling. Questions that can be asked include "Tell me about a specific time when you were feeling depressed?", "Where were you?", "Who were you with?", "What was happening?"

Examples of This Skill in Practice

Context: All patient statements occur after the invitation step (Exercise #3).

Example #1
Patient: I am ready to get to work on my depression.
Therapist: That's great. I love to work with people on their depression. (Criterion 1) Can you share one moment in time when you were feeling depressed? (Criterion 2)

© The Author(s), under exclusive license to Springer Nature Switzerland AG 2023   47
M. Katz et al., *Deliberate Practice of TEAM-CBT*, SpringerBriefs in Psychology,
https://doi.org/10.1007/978-3-031-46019-7_7

Example #2

Patient: I'd like to get to know myself better.

Therapist: Absolutely. I'd love to help you get to know yourself better. (Criterion 1) Can you share one moment in time where you felt like "gosh, I don't really know myself" (Criterion 2)

Example #3

Patient: I really want to get some help with my relationship with my wife.

Therapist: Wonderful. (Criterion 1) Can you tell me about one moment in time when there was a disconnect or conflict with your wife? (Criterion 2)

Now it is your turn: Follow the Exercise Instructions and Skill Criteria (Table 7.1).

After 15 minutes of practice, the patient and therapist switch roles and start over.

Context: All patient statements occur after the invitation step (Exercise #3).

Patient Statement #1 I just need help getting over this anxiety.

Patient Statement #2 I want help with my procrastination.

Patient Statement #3 I need help with my OCD; I can't get anything done.

Patient Statement #4 I need to stop using so much weed!

Patient Statement #5 I can't get myself to do my school homework.

Patient Statement #6 I'm feeling down all the time; nothing gives me any joy.

Table 7.1 Criteria for specificity practice exercise

The therapist improvises a response to each patient statement using the following criteria:
1. Wholeheartedly agree with patients' choice of problem to work on.
2. Ask the patient to select one moment in time when they were experiencing that problem.
Proceed to the next patient statement only when it is too easy for the therapist to meet all criteria.

Patient Statement #7 I can't seem to get control over my phone use and social media surfing. I need to beat this because it is affecting my family, so I am eager to get busy.

Patient Statement #8 I'm so lonely, and I'm having zero success in dating.

Patient Statement #9 I'm bisexual, and I can't talk about it with my mom.

Patient Statement #10 I am ready to get to work and want to figure out how to better my life.

Patient Statement #11 I need help with my wife, she's impossible!

Patient Statement #12 Sometimes I feel like I don't know who I am anymore.

Trainees should attempt to improvise their own responses before reading the example responses (Table 7.2)

Table 7.2 Example therapist responses: specificity

	Patient statements	Example therapist responses
Patient Statement #1	I just need help getting over this anxiety.	That's great. I love to work with people on their anxiety. (Criterion 1) Can you share one moment in time when you were feeling anxious? (Criterion 2)
Patient Statement #2	I want help with my procrastination.	I am so glad to hear that you want to overcome your procrastination. (Criterion 1) Can you describe for me one specific time when you were procrastinatin? What day was that? Where were you at? And what was happening? (Criterion 2)
Patient Statement #3	I need help with my OCD; I can't get anything done.	Absolutely. I'd love to help you with your OCD and help you get things done. (Criterion 1) Can you tell me about one moment in time when you felt the OCD was not letting you get things done? (Criterion 2)
Patient Statement #4	I need to stop using so much weed!	Absolutely, that makes a lot of sense. (Criterion 1) Can you tell me about a moment in time when weed was a problem for you? Where were you and what was happening? (Criterion 2)
Patient Statement #5	I can't get myself to do homework	Absolutely. I'd love to help you with that. (Criterion 1) Can you share one moment in time when you felt you can't get yourself to do homework? (Criterion 2)
Patient Statement #6	I'm feeling down all the time; nothing gives me any joy.	Ugh, how painful to go through life feeling down all the time with no joy. I would love to help you with that. (Criterion 1) Can you share with me a moment in time, and any moment would do, when you felt down and without joy? What were you doing, and where were you? (Criterion 2)

(continued)

Table 7.2 (continued)

	Patient statements	Example therapist responses
Patient Statement #7	I can't seem to get control over my phone use and social media surfing. I need to beat this because it is affecting my family, so I am eager to get busy.	Excellent! Getting control over your phone usage is super important to you, and I am eager to help you with it. (Criterion 1) You mentioned it a number of times when it gets the better of you. Can you select one specific time and tell me what was happening at that moment? (Criterion 2)
Patient Statement #8	I'm so lonely, and I'm having zero success in dating.	Ugh, feeling lonely and getting nowhere with finding a partner are nasty feelings. I'd love to help you with that. (Criterion 1) Can you share one moment in time when you felt lonely and got nowhere with dating? What was happening, and where were you? (Criterion 2)
Patient Statement #9	I'm bisexual, and I can't talk about it with my mom.	Oh, how hard it is that you can't talk about something so important with your mom, I'd love to help you with that. (Criterion 1) Can you share with me a moment in time, and any moment would do, when you felt like you just can't talk about it with her? (Criterion 2)
Patient Statement #10	I am ready to get to work and want to figure out how to better my life.	Wonderful. I am glad to hear you're ready to get to work (Criterion 1) Can you pinpoint for me a specific situation where you were feeling like your life could be better? What were you doing, and who were you with? (Criterion 2)
Patient Statement #11	I need help with my wife, she's impossible!	Absolutely. I'd love to help you with your relationship with your wife. (Criterion 1) Can you tell me about one moment in time when you felt she's impossible? (Criterion 2)
Patient Statement #12	Sometimes I feel like I don't know who I am anymore.	Absolutely. I'd love to help you with that. (Criterion 1) Can you share one moment in time when you were feeling like you just don't know who you are anymore? What was happening at that moment, where were you, and who were you with? (Criterion 2)

Chapter 8
Anticipating Resistance: Conceptualization

Note:This exercise is different from the rest of this book. All other exercises in this book role-play scenarios with a "patient" and "therapist." For this exercise, therapists are not engaged in role-play, but rather reflect and discuss on the topic at hand.

Skill Description

The Conceptualization Step is the third step of agenda setting in TEAM-CBT. It comes after the Invitation and Specificity Steps. This step helps the therapist predict the key resistance factors the patient is likely to have related to the specific problem they chose to work on, thereby setting up the stage for the key next step in therapy: overcoming resistance.

TEAM-CBT proposes that all of the problems therapists can help with can be classified into only four categories: Anxiety, Depression, Relationship Problems, and Habits/Addictions.

Depression problems are characterized by feelings of low self-esteem, inadequacy, guilt, shame, hopelessness, and worthlessness. *Anxiety* problems include worry, panic, fear, and thoughts related to something bad going to happen. *Relationship Problems* involve a disconnect with another person, including conflict in family, work settings, or with intimate partners. Unwanted *Habits and Addictions* cover a range of behaviors that provide some type of short-term pleasure or relief but lead to longer term negative consequences. Examples of Habits/Addictions include procrastination, excessive phone use, gambling, overeating or avoidance of exercise, excessive pornography use, or substance use such as drugs or alcohol.

In TEAM-CBT, as therapists, we look at resistance as inherent and nonpathological, an issue that has to be addressed in order to clear the path for healing. Each conceptualization has two kinds of resistance associated with it: first, Outcome

M. Katz et al., *Deliberate Practice of TEAM-CBT*, SpringerBriefs in Psychology,
https://doi.org/10.1007/978-3-031-46019-7_8

Resistance, or the reasons not to want to reach a seemingly desired goal (Exercise 6A and 6B), and second, Process Resistance, or the reluctance or difficulties with the work necessary to achieve it (Exercise 7A and 7B).

A successful conceptualization step helps the therapist lead the patient toward becoming aware of their "good" reasons not to change and then to melt that resistance away. The conceptualization is often internal and is not discussed in full with the patient. The goal of this exercise is to help you, the therapist, identify the conceptualization category and internalize the following table:

Examples of This Skill in Practice

Context: All patient statements occur after the specificity step (Exercise #4).

Example #1:

Patient: Saturday afternoon, I felt like such a loser and was thinking I was a real failure.

Main conceptualization(s): Depression. (Criterion 1)

What would they have to give up? (Outcome resistance): Give up on your standards for yourself for what is considered a successful life and be willing to love yourself and your life with all of your shortcomings. (Criterion 2)

What work will they have to do to achieve it? (Process resistance): Therapy homework even while feeling unmotivated. (Criterion 3)

Example #2

Patient: Yesterday morning, I just could not pull myself away from checking my Instagram and starting my term paper.

Main conceptualization(s): Habit. (Criterion 1)

What would they have to give up? (Outcome resistance): The joy, instant pleasure, and easy satisfaction of checking Instagram. (Criterion 2)

What work will they have to do to achieve it? (Process resistance): Withdrawal of missing out on the latest posts and reels. Suffering from the craving to open the app on their phone. The boredom and energy drain of working on a term paper. (Criterion 3)

Example #3

Patient: Last week, I got into this argument with my boyfriend, and he left me feeling really bad. I just sat at home and ate a pint of ice cream.

Main conceptualization(s): Relationship Problem, unwanted habit. (Criterion 1)

What would they have to give up? (Outcome resistance):

> **For the relationship problem:** Giving up on the safe emotional distance from your boyfriend and being willing to open up vulnerably to him even if that means being more vulnerable to getting hurt. (Criterion 2)

For the unwanted habit: Give up on a life of easy relief and pleasure, not worrying about what and how much you eat, and get the comfort of it whenever you feel you need it. (Criterion 2)

What work will they have to do to achieve it? (Process resistance):

For the relationship problem: Taking 100% responsibility for the problems in the relationship, not blame the boyfriend at all, and rather see yourself as 100% responsible for the problems in the relationship and for doing the work to fix it. (Criterion 3)

For the unwanted habit: Withdrawal, craving for comfort food, feeling hungry, feeling worse before feeling better, while engaging in new, healthier, less pleasurable eating habits. (Criterion 3)

Now it is your turn: Follow the Exercise Instructions and Skill Criteria (Table 8.1).

After 15 minutes of practice, the patient and therapist switch roles and start over.

Context: All patient statements occur after the specificity step (Exercise #4).

Patient Statement #1 I have an exam on Tuesday, and I get super stressed and worked up, so I cannot concentrate.

Table 8.1 Conceptualization categories and definitions

Conceptualization	Outcome resistance: What would you have to give up if you achieved your goal?	Process resistance: What work will you have to do to achieve your goal?
Depression	Give up on your standards for yourself and the world and instead accept yourself and the world as is.	Therapy homework even while feeling unmotivated.
Anxiety	Give up the protective nature of anxiety, i.e., being prepared and detecting problems early.	Exposure work, i.e., confronting your worst fears.
Relationship problem	Give up on the safe, protective distance from the person you are at odds with.	Taking 100% responsibility for the problems in the relationship and their solution rather than blaming someone else.
Unwanted habit	Give up on a life of easy relief and pleasure.	Withdrawal, craving, and feeling worse before feeling better, while engaging in a new, healthier, less pleasurable behavior.

Patient Statement #2 Fridays after work, I stay at the bar and end up drinking too much.

Patient Statement #3 I wanted to do my therapy homework exercise and go out to the garden, but I kept on feeling: what's the point?

Patient Statement #4 My ex was so difficult to talk to about the weekend plans for the kids on Thursday.

Patient Statement #5 I am trying so hard to diet, but last night, after dinner, I ate a whole bag of chips, family size.

Patient Statement #6 At night, I feel so hopeless and stressed that I will never be able to break free from this depression.

Patient Statement #7 Last night, I was lying in bed and was terrified that my back pain is cancer, my wife and my doctor don't even want to hear about it any more.

Patient Statement #8 My mom and I can never see eye to eye. Yesterday, I just went outside and smoked weed after our argument.

Patient Statement #9 My mom has always been on my case for being heavy. Yesterday, when I came over for dinner, she said, "Sure you need to take seconds?" But she's right, I can only fit into yoga pants now, no professional clothing for me.

Patient Statement #10 Friday I got my paycheck and spent most of it shopping for clothes before paying my rent. Now I am behind, but shopping is the only thing that calms this stress and worry.

Patient Statement #11 I want to quit smoking, so I can be more present with my kids and family, but whenever I cut back, my social life goes out the door. I get awkward and uncomfortable with people, and sometimes irritable with everyone too.

Patient Statement #12 My friends keep pressuring me to hang out and party more, so Saturday I went out. The problem is that I could not stop at two drinks and got totally wasted. My boyfriend got so angry at me when I came home, and now I may lose him.

Trainees should attempt to improvise their own responses before reading the example responses (Table 8.3).

Table 8.2 Criteria for conceptualization practice exercise

Note: This is a reflection and discussion exercise.
Step A. One participant reads the first patient statement.
Step B. The second participant reflects and identifies (Table 8.2):
1. What are the main conceptualization categories the patient's problem fits in.
2. What would the patient have to give up if they achieved their goal? (Outcome resistance)
3. What work will your patient have to do to achieve their goal? (Process resistance)
Step C. Review together the response provided at the end.
Step D. Proceed to the next patient statement.

Table 8.3 Example therapist responses: conceptualization

	Patient statements	Example therapist responses
Patient Statement #1	I have an exam on Tuesday, and I get super stressed and worked up, so I can't concentrate.	**Main conceptualization(s):** Anxiety. (Criterion 1) **What would they have to give up? (Outcome resistance):** Give up the protective nature of anxiety: Being prepared and detecting problems early. (Criterion 2) **What work will they have to do to achieve it? (Process resistance):** Exposure work. Confronting their worst fears, which may involve writing a script, imagining failing miserably on an exam, or setting aside a determined amount of time to study then stopping at that point and sitting with the anxious feeling that will arise when doing something other than studying. (Criterion 3)
Patient Statement #2	On Fridays after work, I stay at the bar and end up drinking too much.	**Main conceptualization(s):** Habit. (Criterion 1) **What would they have to give up? (Outcome resistance):** The joy of enjoying alcohol and socializing at the bar, a life of easy relief and pleasure. (Criterion 2) **What work will they have to do to achieve it? (Process resistance):** Withdrawal, craving, feeling worse before feeling better, while engaging in a new, healthier, less pleasurable behavior that does not involve alcohol. (Criterion 3)
Patient Statement #3	I wanted to do my therapy homework exercise and go out to the garden, but I kept on feeling down and thought: What's the point?	**Main conceptualization(s):** Depression. (Criterion 1) **What would they have to give up? (Outcome resistance):** Give up on their standards for themself/the world. Accept themself and the world as they are. Give up on the idea that they must feel motivated in order to do things. (Criterion 2) **What work will they have to do to achieve it? (Process resistance):** Therapy homework even while feeling unmotivated. (Criterion 3)

(continued)

Table 8.3 (continued)

	Patient statements	Example therapist responses
Patient Statement #4	My ex was so difficult to talk to about the weekend plans for the kids on Thursday.	**Main conceptualization(s):** Relationship Problem. (Criterion 1) **What would they have to give up? (Outcome resistance):** Get closer and connect with the person she is at odds with. Give up on the safe distance from the ex. (Criterion 2) **What work will they have to do to achieve it? (Process resistance):** Taking 100% responsibility for the problems in the relationship and their solutions, rather than blaming someone else. (Criterion 3)
Patient Statement #5	I'm trying so hard to diet, but last night, after dinner, I ate a whole bag of chips, family size.	**Main conceptualization(s):** Habit. (Criterion 1) **What would they have to give up? (Outcome resistance):** The simple and instant pleasure and satisfaction of enjoying delicious chips in the evening. (Criterion 2) **What work will they have to do to achieve it? (Process resistance):** Withdrawal, craving, feeling worse before feeling better, while engaging in a new, healthier, less pleasurable behavior, including eating bland and boring veggies and doing a workout in the evening. (Criterion 3)
Patient Statement #6	At night, I feel so hopeless, and I get stressed that I will never be able to break free from this depression	**Main conceptualization(s):** Depression. (Criterion 1) **What would they have to give up? (Outcome resistance):** Give up hopelessness, accept themself and the world as they are. (Criterion 2) **What work will they have to do to achieve it? (Process resistance):** Do the work necessary to overcome hopelessness and depression, including therapy homework even while feeling unmotivated. (Criterion 3)
Patient Statement #7	Last night, I was lying in bed and was terrified that my back pain is cancer. My wife and my doctor don't even want to hear about it anymore.	**Main conceptualization(s):** Anxiety. (Criterion 1) **What would they have to give up? (Outcome resistance):** Give up the protective nature of anxiety, including being prepared and detecting problems early. Give up on the vigilance of staying on top of every health concern. (Criterion 2) **What work will they have to do to achieve it? (Process resistance):** Exposure work. Confronting their worst fears. This might involve imaginal exposure, refraining from researching symptoms, or refraining from checking in with their wife and doctor. (Criterion 3)

(continued)

Table 8.3 (continued)

	Patient statements	Example therapist responses
Patient Statement #8	My mom and I can never see eye to eye. Yesterday, I just went outside and smoked weed after our argument.	**Main conceptualization(s):** Relationship Problem, Unwanted habit. (Criterion 1) **What would they have to give up? (Outcome resistance):** **For the relationship problem:** Get closer and more connected and intimate with their mom. (Criterion 2) **For unwanted habit:** Give up on the joy and relief and the life of easy relief and pleasure through smoking marijuana. (Criterion 2) **What work will they have to do to achieve it? (Process resistance):** **For the relationship problem:** Taking 100% responsibility for the problems in the relationship and their solutions such as working on communication with mom and seeing the world from where she stands, rather than blaming others. (Criterion 3) **For unwanted habit:** Withdrawal, craving, feeling worse before feeling better, while engaging in a new, healthier, less pleasurable behavior than smoking marijuana. (Criterion 3)
Patient Statement #9	My mom has always been on my case for being heavy. Yesterday, when I came over for dinner she said, "Sure you need to take seconds?" But she's right, I can only fit into yoga pants now, no professional clothing for me.	**Main conceptualization(s):** Relationship Problem, Unwanted habit. (Criterion 1) **What would they have to give up? (Outcome resistance):** **For the relationship problem:** Give up on the safe distance from mom and the urge to get defensive with her or avoid her. (Criterion 2) **For the unwanted habit:** Give up on a life of easy relief and pleasure that involves enjoying seconds at dinner and making the most of the delicious meal she always makes. (Criterion 2) **What work will they have to do to achieve it? (Process resistance):** **For the relationship problem:** Taking 100% responsibility for the problems in the relationship, rather than blaming others. (Criterion 3) **For the unwanted habit:** Withdrawal, craving, feeling worse before feeling better, while engaging in a new, healthier, less pleasurable behavior. Taking smaller portions and getting up from the table after the first serving. Going for walks with mom rather than sitting around the table eating and chatting. (Criterion 3)

(continued)

Table 8.3 (continued)

	Patient statements	Example therapist responses
Patient Statement #10	Friday, I got my paycheck and spent most of it shopping for clothes before paying my rent. Now I am behind but shopping is the only thing that calms this stress and worry.	**Main conceptualization(s):** Unwanted habit, Anxiety. (Criterion 1) **What would they have to give up? (Outcome resistance):** **For the unwanted habit:** Give up on shopping as a way for relief and pleasure. (Criterion 2) **For anxiety:** Give up the protective and motivating nature of anxiety including being prepared and taking action. (Criterion 2) **What work will they have to do to achieve it? (Process resistance):** **For the unwanted habit:** Withdrawal, craving, feeling worse before feeling better, while engaging in a new, healthier, less pleasurable behavior. (Criterion 3) **For anxiety:** Exposure work including confronting your worst fears. (Criterion 3)
Patient Statement #11	I want to quit smoking, so I can be more present with my kids and family, but whenever I cut back, my social life goes out the door. I get awkward and uncomfortable with people, and sometimes irritable with everyone too.	**Main conceptualization(s):** Unwanted habit, Anxiety. (Criterion 1) **What would they have to give up? (Outcome resistance):** **For the unwanted habit:** Give up on the easy relief and pleasure of lighting up and having a smoke. (Criterion 2) **For Anxiety:** Give up the protective nature of anxiety: Preventing those awkward and uncomfortable moments. (Criterion 2) **For the relationship problem:** Give up on the safe distance from friends and family and the protection from their vulnerability of seeing the patient as they are. (Criterion 2) **What work will they have to do to achieve it? (Process resistance):** **For the unwanted habit:** Withdrawals from smoking and having to endure the craving, feeling worse and perhaps more irritable before feeling better. Engaging in a new healthier, less pleasurable behavior such as exercise or meditation whenever the urge to smoke arises. (Criterion 3) **For Anxiety:** Exposure work, including confronting your worst fears. Facing the awkward and uncomfortable nature of learning social and communication skills with friends and family. (Criterion 3) **For the relationship problem:** Taking 100% responsibility for the problems in the relationships and working hard to learn new ways to engage and communicate, rather than blame others. (Criterion 3)

(continued)

Table 8.3 (continued)

	Patient statements	Example therapist responses
Patient Statement #12	My friends keep pressuring me to hang out and party more, so Saturday I went out. The problem is that I could not stop at two drinks and got totally wasted. My boyfriend got so angry at me when I came home, and now I may lose him.	**Main conceptualization(s):** Relationship, Unwanted habit, Anxiety. (Criterion 1) **What would they have to give up? (Outcome resistance):** **For the relationship problem:** Connect vulnerably with the boyfriend and pressuring friends, give up on the safe distance from other people. (Criterion 2) **For the unwanted habit:** Give up on the joy and social lubricant aspects of alcohol, give up on a life of easy relief and pleasure. (Criterion 2) **For Anxiety:** Give up the protective and motivating nature of anxiety. Be prepared for being alone, without a boyfriend. Have motivation to improve the relationship. (Criterion 2) **What work will they have to do to achieve it? (Process resistance):** **For the relationship problem:** Taking 100% responsibility for the problems in the relationships and their solutions such as improving communication, learn to vulnerably communicate your anger and guilt feelings rather than blame others. (Criterion 3) **For the unwanted habit:** Withdrawal, craving, feeling worse before feeling better, while engaging in a new, healthier, less pleasurable behavior than drinking. (Criterion 3) **For Anxiety:** Exposure work including confronting your worst fears about being alone or in conflict. (Criterion 3)

(continued)

Chapter 9
Uncovering Good Reasons Not to Change: Magic Button Step 1

Skill Description

As therapists, we address outcome resistance and use the magic button question as the fourth step in agenda setting. This happens only after an invitation is accepted (Chap. 6), and we have used specificity (Chap. 7) and conceptualization (Chap. 8) to clearly delineate the problem. "Outcome resistance" refers to all the good and positive reasons a person may not want to overcome an identified problem or get relief from their negative feelings or unwanted behaviors. To overcome the obstacles toward a wanted change, the patient must first bring the good reasons to cling to their symptoms into their conscious awareness, and then confront them and melt them away. Invariably, they will find that upsetting emotions or "negative" behaviors reveal admirable core values about themselves. When a patient asks us for help and relief from their pain and unwanted feelings, the therapist will need to resist a powerful urge to offer them help right away. If we fall for the urge and rush to "help" without first confronting the good reasons not to change, our efforts will fall flat and even the cleverest cognitive behavioral techniques will fail. We often find that the bulk of therapy is spent using Outcome Resistance techniques. The Magic Button question is the first one of several other Outcome Resistance methods that follow.

This is the structure to present the Magic Button question: "If, with a push of a button, all of your anxiety (for example) will instantly disappear, completely and forever, would you push that button?" Importantly, the therapist must always include the result from pushing the magic button, i.e., the complete and immediate elimination of symptoms.

The Magic Button question helps stimulate the patient's thinking toward aspects they usually do not think positively about what is good and great about their symptoms, such as feeling anxious, depressed, angry, procrastinating, or about addictions. It is presented to invite our patients to think carefully about the outcome or result of recovery. This sets up a deeper investigation of what will be lost with full recovery including the function the symptom serves and what values it reveals about our patient.

Examples of This Skill in Practice

Context: All patient statements occur after the conceptualization step (Exercise #5).

Example #1
Patient: I hate that I can't fit into any of my clothes. I just want to feel better about who I am.
Therapist: So, if we had a magic button right in front of us, and with a push of that button, you'd feel great about yourself instantly. Would you push that button?

Example #2
Patient: I feel so down all the time and need to get out of this depression.
Therapist: If we had a magic button on the desk right in front of you and you pushed it, instantly you would feel relief from your depression. Would you push that button?

Example #3
Patient: I'm anxious all the time.
Therapist: So, if we had a magic button right in front of us, and with a push of that button, you'd feel no more anxiety. Would you push that button?

> **Now it is your turn: Follow the Exercise Instructions and Skill Criteria (Table 9.1).**

> **After 15 minutes of practice, the patient and therapist switch roles and start over.**

Table 9.1 Criteria for magic button Part 1 practice exercise

The therapist improvises a response to each patient statement using the following criteria:
1. Present the "magic button" question. (Must include the words "magic button" and present the result from pushing the magic button, i.e., the complete and immediate elimination of symptoms.)
2. The presentation should be clear and succinct.
Proceed to the next patient statement <u>only</u> when it is too easy for the therapist to meet all criteria.

Context: All patient statements occur after the conceptualization step (Exercise 5).

Patient Statement #1 I just want to feel better about who I am even if I am overweight.

Patient Statement #2 I keep having this thought that I am a failure. I feel so inadequate, and I want to be free from it.

Patient Statement #3 I want to feel more confident when I meet new people. I am always so self-conscious and anxious.

Patient Statement #4 I want to overcome my crippling anxiety around people.

Patient Statement #5 I need to stop smoking weed.

Patient Statement #6 I need to stop procrastinating so much and do my schoolwork.

Patient Statement #7 I need to stop drinking.

Patient Statement #8 I need to get my sleep schedule in order. I'm up at night and asleep till the afternoon.

Patient Statement #9 I want to have a better relationship with my ex-wife.

Patient Statement #10 I keep losing my temper, and I need to get my anger under control.

Patient Statement #11 I want to date more and find a long-term relationship.

Patient Statement #12 I do want help to overcome this hopelessness. It is so hard.

Trainees should attempt to improvise their own responses before reading the example responses (Table 9.2).

Table 9.2 Example therapist responses: magic button Part1

	Patient statements	Example therapist responses
Patient Statement #1	I just want to feel better about who I am even if I am overweight.	Imagine that we have a magic button on the desk in front of you. If you push that button, instantly you will feel great about yourself. Would you push that button?
Patient Statement #2	I keep having this thought that I am a failure. I feel so inadequate, and I want to be free from it.	So if we had a magic button right in front of us here, and with a push of that button, you'd never feel the least bit inadequate or a sense of failure at all. Would you push that button?
Patient Statement #3	I want to feel more confident when I meet new people. I am always so self-conscious and anxious.	If we had a magic button and you pushed it right now, you would be free from your anxiety and self-consciousness, as well as feel tremendous confidence in meeting new people. Would you push that button?
Patient Statement #4	I want to overcome my crippling anxiety around people.	So if we had a magic button right in front of us here, with a push of a magic button, you could make all of your anxiety around people completely vanish. Would you push that button?
Patient Statement #5	I need to stop smoking weed.	Let's imagine we have a magic button right there in front of us. If you push that button, you will be completely free from your weed-smoking habit. Would you push that button?
Patient Statement #6	I need to stop procrastinating so much and do my schoolwork.	So if we had a magic button right in front of us here, and with a push of a magic button, you would never procrastinate at all and would always immediately complete all of your schoolwork with no delay. Would you push that button?
Patient Statement #7	I need to stop drinking.	Let's imagine we have a magic button on the desk right in front of you. If you push that button, drinking will no longer be a part of your life. You will be totally free from it. Would you push that button?
Patient Statement #8	I need to get my sleep schedule in order. I'm up at night and asleep till the afternoon.	So if we had a magic button in front of us, and with a push of that button, you'd always go to sleep at the same time at night and get out of bed at the same earlier time in the morning. Would you push that button?
Patient Statement #9	I want to have a better relationship with my ex-wife.	Imagine I offered you a magic button, and if you pushed, it instantly you would have a great relationship with your ex-wife. Would you push that button?
Patient Statement #10	I keep losing my temper, and I need to get my anger under control.	Now, if there was a magic button in front of you, and with a push of that button, you'd never feel angry again, no matter what. Would you push that button?

(continued)

Table 9.2 (continued)

	Patient statements	Example therapist responses
Patient Statement #11	I want to date more and find a long-term relationship.	Let's imagine we have a magic button right there in front of you. If you pushed that button, you would instantly feel confident and motivated to put yourself out there and date more. Would you press that button?
Patient Statement #12	I do want help to overcome this hopelessness. It is so hard.	If we had a magic button in front of us, and with a push of that button, all of your hopelessness would completely vanish, and you would only feel hopeful about everything all the time. Would you push that button?

Chapter 10
Uncovering Good Reasons Not to Change: Magic Button Step 2

Skill Description

After the therapist presents the magic button, patients usually respond by enthusiastically wanting to push it. Other times, they hesitate. Either way, our response is the same: to slow down and help them think about the positive things their symptoms show about them as human beings, and the benefits their particular suffering brings to their lives. Our goal is to help the patient bring to conscious awareness the reasons they may not want to change: what is beautiful, good, and great about their symptoms. For example:

- Feeling anxious can help motivate action, keep us vigilant to danger, and protect us from the consequences of unwise decisions.
- Feelings of guilt and shame can help us learn from mistakes, reveal a high moral standard, and show that we are willing to take responsibility for our actions.
- Habits and addictions such as drinking or overeating provide short-term pleasure or relief.

This is a counterintuitive position for both the therapist and the patient to be in. Rather than argue for the elimination of depression/anxiety/unwanted habits/relationship difficulties, the therapist argues for seeing the good in the continuation of the suffering. Paradoxically, this allows our patients to be able to let go of their resistance to change. It also allows us, the therapist, to align with their resistance and for the patient to take on the role of arguing for change.[1]

In this exercise, the therapist will practice fleshing out the outcome resistance reasons internal to the patient. The therapist starts by affirming the patient's choice

---

[1] Typically, both therapist and patient then write down a list of the good and positive reasons not to change. Later, the therapist uses the list to confront the patient with those reasons not to change, often using the Externalization of Resistance technique, a technique similar to Externalization of Voices, which we will cover in a later chapter.

© The Author(s), under exclusive license to Springer Nature Switzerland AG 2023
M. Katz et al., *Deliberate Practice of TEAM-CBT*, SpringerBriefs in Psychology,
https://doi.org/10.1007/978-3-031-46019-7_10

regarding the magic button question (e.g., "It makes total sense that you'd want to push this button!"). The therapist then immediately follows this by inviting the patient to slow down (e.g., "Hold on, let's think about this."). Finally, the therapist directs the patient to consider the positive benefits they would lose if all of their depression/anxiety/unwanted habits/relationship difficulties vanished with the push of the button (e.g., "What would you stand to lose if you were to push that button?") and/or directs the patient to consider some of the beautiful values their difficulties show about them (e.g., "What are the good things feeling depressed/anxious/having this relationship difficulty/unwanted habit say about you?").

Examples of This Skill in Practice

Context: All patient statements occur right after presenting the Magic Button question (Exercise #6A).

Example #1
Patient: Absolutely. Of course, I'd push that button and feel great about myself.
Therapist: I agree, but let's hold on and think about this. (Criterion 1) What would you stand to lose if you pushed that button (Criterion 2), and what does it reveal about your value system that is admirable? (Criterion 3)

Example #2
Patient: Of course, I would love to push that button and be free from depression and feeling so down all the time.
Therapist: It does sound good, doesn't it? At the same time, let's pause for a minute (Criterion 1) and consider what would be lost if we pushed that button. There are some important benefits to feeling depressed (Criterion 2), and it reveals some values you hold that are admirable. (Criterion 3)

Example #3
Patient: Of course, I would love to push that button and be rid of this anxiety.
Therapist: I am right with you there, but let's hang on for a second and think about it. (Criterion 1) There are some tremendous benefits to feeling anxious (Criterion 2), and your anxiety shows some wonderful things about you and your values. (Criterion 3) Can we think about those together? (Criterion 1)

Now it is your turn: Follow the Exercise Instructions and Skill Criteria (Table 10.1).

After 15 minutes of practice, the patient and therapist switch roles and start over.

Table 10.1 Criteria for magic button Part 2 practice exercise

The therapist improvises a response to each patient statement using the following criteria:

1. Affirm the patient's choice, then direct the patient to pause.

2. Direct the patient to consider the positive benefits they would lose if all of their depression/anxiety/unwanted habits/relationship difficulties would vanish with the push of a button.

3. Direct the patient to consider some of the *beautiful values* their depression/anxiety/ unwanted habits/relationship difficulties show about them.

Proceed to the next patient statement only when it is too easy for the therapist to meet all criteria.

Context: All patient statements occur right after presenting the Magic Button question (Exercise 6A).

Patient Statement #1 For sure, I would push that button if it meant feeling great about myself.

Patient Statement #2 Yes, I would push that button to get rid of feeling inadequate and like a failure.

Patient Statement #3 Of course. In a heartbeat, I would push that button to be free from my anxiety and self-consciousness and feel tremendous confidence in meeting new people.

Patient Statement #4 No question. I would push that button if it meant all of my anxiety around people completely vanished.

Patient Statement #5 Of course. I want to push that button to be free from smoking weed.

Patient Statement #6 I would definitely push that button if it meant I was over procrastinating with my schoolwork.

Patient Statement #7 Yes, I will push that button right now to be done with drinking.

Patient Statement #8 For sure. Pushing the button sounds great if it means I get my sleep schedule on track.

Patient Statement #9 Well, I don't want to get back together with her, but if it meant that we could at least get along for the kids' sake, then yes, I would push it.

Patient Statement #10 Of course, I would push that button if it meant my anger was gone and I would no longer lose my temper.

Patient Statement #11 I am not sure if I would push it. To instantly feel confident and motivated to put myself out there and date more sounds enticing, but scary too.

Patient Statement #12 That sounds too good to be true, but I would definitely push it to have this hopelessness disappear.

Trainees should attempt to improvise their own responses before reading the example responses (Table 10.2).

Table 10.2 Example therapist responses: magic button Part 2

	Patient statements	Example therapist responses
Patient statement #1	For sure, I would push that button if it meant feeling great about myself.	Absolutely! There's nothing more I wish for you than to feel great about yourself. But still, hold on, let's think about it together. (Criterion 1) What would you stand to lose if you pushed the button and became 100% self-assured all the time? (Criterion 2) What are the good things it says about you that you don't feel 100% self-assured all the time? (Criterion 3)
Patient Statement #2	Yes, I would push that button to get rid of feeling inadequate and like a failure.	Yeah, that sounds good, doesn't it. But let's pause for a moment to consider (Criterion 1) together what will be lost if we push that button. There are many wonderful benefits to feelings this way. (Criterion 2) and they point to some things you really value. (Criterion 3)
Patient statement #3	Of course. In a heartbeat, I would push that button to be free from my anxiety and self-consciousness and feel tremendous confidence in meeting new people.	Makes perfect sense! But let's pause here and consider this for a moment, (Criterion 1) what are the good things feeling anxious and self-conscious say about you? What are the values feeling anxious shows you have? (Criterion 3) How might feeling anxious help you? (Criterion 2)
Patient statement #4	No question. I would push that button if it meant all of my anxiety around people completely vanished.	For sure, I would too. At the same time, I am feeling a little hesitant about having you push that button and think we should hold and consider (Criterion 1) what might be lost. Can you think of any benefits or advantages to feeling anxious (Criterion 2), and what feeling anxious say about you and your values that is awesome and wonderful? (Criterion 3)
Patient Statement #5	Of course, I want to push that button to be free from smoking weed.	I can see that, but let's slow down here. (Criterion 1) Let's consider: What does Marijuana do for you that you'd lose if you'd stopped smoking? (Criterion 2) What are the positive things it says about you that you smoke weed from time to time? (Criterion 3)
Patient statement #6	Yes, I would push that button so I can finally be free from procrastinating and be able to complete all of my schoolwork with no delay.	I totally agree with you. But let's hang on for a second and consider (Criterion 1) what you would be giving up if you pushed that button. Let's think together about some of the benefits of procrastination (Criterion 2) and what it shows about the things you value that are important. (Criterion 3)

(continued)

Table 10.2 (continued)

	Patient statements	Example therapist responses
Patient statement #7	Definitely. Pushing the button sounds great if it means I get my sleep schedule on track.	That would be great, wouldn't it? Absolutely, but let's hold on here. (Criterion 1) Let's think together about the benefits of not having a super strict sleep schedule? (Criterion 2) What are the good things it says about you and your values as a person that you don't have a super strict sleep schedule? (Criterion 3)
Patient statement #8	For sure. Pushing the button sounds great if it means I get my sleep schedule on track.	Agreed. (Criterion 1) But let's wait before we rush into it and explore the impact of pushing that button. We may be losing some important benefits to hanging on to your current sleep routine (Criterion 2)
Patient statement #9	Well, I don't want to get back together with my ex-wife, but if pushing the button meant that we could get along better for the kids' sake, then yes, I would push it.	Yeah, you'd do anything for your kids! That's really beautiful about you. But hold on, let's think about it. (Criterion 1) Would you really want to have a closer, more emotionally intimate relationship with your ex-wife? You've worked hard at setting some boundaries with her. What do you stand to lose if you were emotionally close to her again? (Criterion 2) Let's think, what are the good things it says about you as a person that you keep your distance from her. (Criterion 3)
Patient statement #10	Of course, I would push that button if it meant my anger was gone and I would no longer lose my temper.	That is true, and I am right with you. (Criterion 1) At the same time, I think we should pause for a minute and consider what your anger says about you that is actually wonderful and awesome, about the things you value that are important. (Criterion 3) Let us also look at how your anger may be a real asset to you (Criterion 2)
Patient statement #11	I am not sure if I would push it. To instantly feel confident and motivated to put myself out there and date more sounds enticing, but scary too.	That is absolutely true, and I am right with you. I am not sure I would push it either. (Criterion 1) Let's explore together some of the things you would lose if you push that button (Criterion 2) and what your upsetting thoughts and emotions reveal about you that is admirable and wonderful. (Criterion 3)
Patient statement #12	That sounds too good to be true, but I would definitely push it to have this hopelessness disappear.	I agree. (Criterion 1) This may sound strange, but we may want to hold on for a minute before we jump in and push that button. There may be some real benefits to feeling hopeless that you would lose (Criterion 2) and it shows some wonderful things about your character and what you value. Let's think together about what those are. (Criterion 3)

Chapter 11
Boosting Motivation: Dangling the Carrot

Skill Description

Addressing Process Resistance is the last step in the five sequential steps of melting away resistance and boosting motivation with TEAM-CBT. It comes only after we, the therapist, address Outcome Resistance, as outlined in exercises 6A and 6B. Once we feel convinced that the patient has confronted all that they stand to lose if they bring about change, they turn to Process Resistance – the resistance to *doing the work* necessary in order to achieve that change. A good result of the Process Resistance step in therapy is when the patient states clearly that they are eager and willing to do whatever it takes in order to bring about the desired change.

The therapist's stance is paradoxical in nature. While we do not advocate for change, we are confident that complete change is possible, but only with the hefty price of hard work. We do not underestimate or overestimate the work and its difficulty. We state clearly what it would entail in order to recover and ask the patient whether they would like to do that work, even though it will be quite difficult. The therapist also clarifies that there are no guarantees of success and that we would not hold it against them, and would love them just the same, whether they do the work or not.

Process Resistance is addressed with a sequence of techniques, namely, Dangling the Carrot, Issuing the Gentle Ultimatum, Fallback Position, and Sitting with Open Hands.[1]

This exercise focuses on the first key technique to address Process Resistance: *Dangling the Carrot*. The purpose of this technique is to instill hope in the patient.

---

[1] A common mistake therapists make is to fail to dangle the carrot before issuing the ultimatum (Exercise 7B). This invariably results in the patient feeling hopelessness and rejection, which can serve as a reminder to go back and issue the dangling the carrot technique.

In order to do that, the therapist names three elements that may make the work of therapy enticing:

1. Complete relief or removal of symptoms
2. The excitement of working together in collaboration
3. Obtaining skills and tools the patient can use for the rest of their life

Examples of This Skill in Practice

Example #1
Patient: Yes, I want to control my alcohol abuse.
Therapist: Absolutely! I'd be delighted to work with you (Criterion 1) and help you get complete control over the alcohol use. (Criterion 2) There are many powerful skills and techniques I'd be eager to explore with you, which you could then use for the rest of your life. (Criterion 3)

Example #2
Patient: I want to overcome my social anxiety, but I am not sure about doing exposure work.
Therapist: Excellent, working with anxiety is one of my favorite things. (Criterion 1) I have worked with a lot of people who have experienced the relief from anxiety you are going for and I am confident we can deliver that for you too. (Criterion 2) I have a host of incredible tools and techniques we can learn and use to get that relief long term. (Criterion 3)

Example #3
Patient: I need to overcome depression, but I don't have the motivation to do therapy homework right now.
Therapist: Absolutely, I'm eager to work with you (Criterion 1) and help you overcome this depression. (Criterion 2) We have many tools to work with and teach you, which can help tremendously. (Criterion 3)

Now it is your turn: Follow the Exercise Instructions and Skill Criteria (Table 11.1).

After 15 minutes of practice, the patient and therapist switch roles and start over.

Patient Statement #1 I am tired of feeling this much anxiety and need to get some relief from it.

Table 11.1 Criteria for dangling the carrot practice exercise

The therapist improvises a response to each patient statement using the following criteria:
1. Express excitement about the opportunity to work together.
2. State clearly that complete elimination of symptoms is possible.
3. Convey that there are many powerful skills and tools the patient can learn and use for the rest of their life.
Proceed to the next patient statement only when it is too easy for the therapist to meet all criteria.

Patient Statement #2 I want to figure out the communication in my relationship, but my partner doesn't ever listen.

Patient Statement #3 I have tried everything to manage my anxiety, nothing seems to last.

Patient Statement #4 I just can't seem to get around to doing my taxes.

Patient Statement #5 The problem is my wife. She really needs to change the way she talks to me.

Patient Statement #6 I don't like using forms, and surveys. They are too technical.

Patient Statement #7 First I need to sleep better, then I can quit smoking pot.

Patient Statement #8 I'm not the type who does homework.

Patient Statement #9 First, I need to get over this depression, then I'll feel that life is worth living and won't contemplate suicide.

Patient Statement #10 I can't keep going with this depression and feeling so hopeless. Nothing is going to work.

Patient Statement #11 The real problem isn't my drinking; it's just that I'm depressed. I could quit anytime, and I'm just self-medicating the depression.

Patient Statement #12 I am the one doing all the work in this relationship, but I am not ready to give up on her yet. She just needs to change the way she talks to me.

Trainees should attempt to improvise their own responses before reading the example responses. (Table 11.2).

Table 11.2 Example therapist responses: dangling the carrot

	Patient statement	Example therapist response
Patient statement #1	I am tired of feeling this much anxiety and need to get some relief from it.	Absolutely. I'd be delighted to work with you to overcome anxiety. (Criterion 1) Overcoming anxiety (Criterion 2) is one of my favorite things to do with my patients and I have many powerful skills and tools to show and teach you, which will serve you now and in the future. (Criterion 3)
Patient statement #2	I want to figure out the communication in my relationship but my partner doesn't ever listen.	It would be great to work with you to figure out the communication in your relationship. (Criterion 1) We have a number of very powerful strategies and tools that can bring about significant transformation in relationships (Criterion 2) and lead to the closeness with your partner that you want. (Criterion 3)
Patient statement #3	I have tried everything to manage my anxiety, nothing seems to last.	I'd be delighted to work with you on that every step of the way. (Criterion 1) Anxiety disorders can be awful, yet they can be completely overcome (Criterion 2) using the many powerful tools and techniques we now have against them. The neat thing is that once we find the tools that work for you, you'll be able to make use of them whenever you need to. (Criterion 3)
Patient statement #4	I just can't seem to get around to doing my taxes.	One of my favorite things is working with people to overcome the barriers that get in the way of our goals like getting taxes done. I would love to show you (Criterion 1) how to get you out of this rut for good (Criterion 2) I have a host of amazing tools and strategies we can utilize. (Criterion 3)
Patient statement #5	The problem is my wife. She really needs to change the way she talks to me.	I'd love to work with you (Criterion 1) and help you change the relationship with your wife so you can truly live happily ever after. (Criterion 2) There are awesome communication skills and numerous other techniques we could employ towards that; tools that will help you with your wife and really with all other relationships as well going forward. (Criterion 3)
Patient statement #6	I want to feel better but I don't like using forms, and surveys. They are too technical.	I would love to work with you (Criterion #1) to show you how to feel better and be completely free from this depression and anxiety you have been experiencing. (Criterion 2) There are a variety of incredible strategies and tools we can explore that are effective in bringing about the long-term change in mood you desire. (Criterion 3)
Patient statement #7	First, I need to sleep better, then I can quit smoking pot.	I'd be delighted to work with you and get you to sleep well! (Criterion 1) While sleep problems can feel frustrating and daunting they can be completely overcome (Criterion 2) with good therapy, tools, and techniques I can show you that will serve you now and for the rest of your life. (Criterion 3)

(continued)

Table 11.2 (continued)

	Patient statement	Example therapist response
Patient statement #8	I'm not the type that does homework, but I need something to help me be free from this anxiety.	Working with anxiety is one of my favorite things and I would love to work with you on it. (Criterion 1) I have seen full and complete recovery for many of my patients and I am confident this is possible for you too. (Criterion 2) I have many powerful and effective tools that can bring about the relief you are looking for. (Criterion 3)
Patient statement #9	First, I need to get over this depression, then I'll feel that life is worth living and won't contemplate suicide.	Makes complete sense. I'd love to work with you side by side untill you overcome this depression completely. (Criteria 1 and 2) There are numerous tools and techniques we can use to get you there and keep you there. You'll be able to use them now and any time you're feeling pulled down by depression in the future too. (Criterion 3)
Patient statement #10	I can't keep going with this depression and feeling so hopeless. Nothing is going to work.	Working with people with depression is something I consider a real privilege. It would be a pleasure to support you in your journey. (Criterion 1) This may sound optimistic, but I have experienced myself and witnessed in others that a full and lasting recovery from depression is possible. (Criterion 2) The tools and techniques we now have available are incredible and I am confident we can get you to the place of joy and self-esteem that you have longed for. (Criterion 3)
Patient statement #11	The real problem isn't my drinking, it's just that I'm depressed, I could quit anytime and I'm just self-medicating the depression.	There's little that would make me happier than to work with you to overcome this depression you've been self-medicating. (Criteria 1 and 2) There's no doubt in mind you could completely overcome it (Criterion 2) and the cool thing is that you'll be able to use the powerful tools and techniques I can show you not only now but for the rest of your life whenever you're feeling down. (Criterion 3)
Patient statement #12	I am the one doing all the work in this relationship, but I am not ready to give up on her yet. She just needs to change the way she talks to me.	Relationship work is challenging but incredibly rewarding, and it would be amazing to work with you to bring about the change you are hoping for. (Criterion 1) Obtaining that closeness, connection, and intimacy with your partner is possible with the powerful new tools, techniques, and strategies that we have. (Criteria 2 and 3)

Chapter 12
Making the Patient Accountable: Issuing the Gentle Ultimatum

Skill Description

The goal of the gentle ultimatum is to make the patient aware of what is required of them in order to reach their goal and to pass the responsibility for that work squarely on to their shoulders without judgment on our part if they choose not to do so and rather work toward a different goal. It typically follows Outcome Resistance (see Chaps. 9 and 10) and 6B) and is usually coupled with Dangling the Carrot (Chap. 11).

This is one of the hardest TEAM-CBT techniques for therapists to do, as it is typically difficult for therapists to set boundaries and make demands, let alone issue an ultimatum to patients! When done well, the patient leaves the conversation with hope and a clear understanding of what it would take for them to reach their goal, while also feeling that their therapist cares about them and is committed to their success. Therapists leave the conversation feeling aligned with their patient and relieved, knowing that they did not set their patient with false expectations and that they are not expected to miraculously do things that cannot typically be done in therapy such as overcoming anxiety without exposure, dealing with substance use without sobriety, improving relationship problems without accountability and eliminating blame, or overcoming depression without therapy homework, activation, etc.

In order to do this technique well, therapists will need to have a very clear understanding of what is the nature of the work required from the patient to overcome each kind of therapy problem. When starting off, it is recommended to have the Process Resistance part of the Conceptualization table (See Chap. 8) as a reminder.

Dangling the Carrot (Chap. 11) and the Gentle Ultimatum techniques are typically a one-two punch duo. Therapists start with the Carrot to instill hope and motivation, followed by the Gentle Ultimatum that states clearly what will be required of the patients in order to reach their specific goal, without minimizing its difficulty.

© The Author(s), under exclusive license to Springer Nature Switzerland AG 2023 79
M. Katz et al., *Deliberate Practice of TEAM-CBT*, SpringerBriefs in Psychology,
https://doi.org/10.1007/978-3-031-46019-7_12

This is done while conveying a preference to work together and complete respect for the patient's option not to do so but rather to focus on a different goal if they wish.

Examples of This Skill in Practice

Example #1
Patient: I want to control my alcohol abuse.

Therapist: That sounds great, but before we jump in, I want to be clear about what that will require. I will be asking you to do written daily homework, get a support system set up including your friends and family, and be willing to deprive yourself of the pleasure of drinking. (Criterion 1) That is a lot to ask, (Criterion 2) but I don't know how to help people overcome alcohol abuse without it. (Criterion 3) While I would love to work with you, (Criterion 4) I fully support your decision if you decide this is not the approach for you. (Criterion 5)

Example #2
Patient: I want to overcome my social anxiety, but I am not sure about doing exposure work.

Therapist: I completely understand that exposure work is not for everybody, and it may not be worth it to you (Criterion 5) to go through something so difficult (Criterion 2) just to overcome your anxiety. I have complete respect for that. (Criterion 5) The problem is that I don't know how to help people overcome their anxiety without doing exposure. (Criterion 3) Don't get me wrong, I'd love to work with you and help you completely overcome your anxiety, (Criterion 4) but it would require confronting and experiencing things you normally wouldn't do. First with me and then without me, (Criterion 1) and it could be quite hard. (Criterion 2) Perhaps there's something else you'd like us to work on other than anxiety that doesn't require exposure? (Criterion 5)

Example #3
Patient: I need to overcome depression, but I don't have the motivation to do therapy homework right now.

    Therapist: I'm so sorry, I would love to work with you, (Criterion 4) I just don't know how to help people overcome depression without doing a lot of therapy homework (Criteria 2 and 3) including reading, paper and pencil exercises to challenge your negative thoughts, and other techniques first with me and then on your own. (Criterion 1) I would hate to see you go, but of course I'd be willing to refer you to therapists who don't assign homework as part of their treatment. What would you prefer? (Criterion 5)

Now it is your turn: Follow the Exercise Instructions and Skill Criteria (Table 12.1).

Table 12.1 Criteria for gentle ultimatum practice exercise

The therapist improvises a response to each patient statement using the following criteria:
1. **State clearly what is needed in order to recover. (Gentle Ultimatum)**
2. **Convey that the work required is hard.**
3. **State "I don't know how to help people overcome [problem] without [required work]."**
4. **Convey excitement about working together. (Dangling the Carrot)**
5. **Convey respect in fully supporting any direction the patient decides. (Sitting with Open Hand)**

Proceed to the next patient statement only when it is too easy for the therapist to meet all criteria.

After 15 minutes of practice, the patient and therapist switch roles and start over.

For these next statements, the patient is pleasant and receptive.

Patient Statement #1 I am tired of feeling this much anxiety and need to get some relief from it.

Patient Statement #2 I want to figure out the communication in my relationship, but my partner doesn't ever listen.

Patient Statement #3 I have tried everything to manage my anxiety, nothing seems to last.

Patient Statement #4 I just can't seem to get around to doing my taxes.

For these next statements, the patient is somewhat receptive and somewhat open to getting to work.

Patient Statement #5 The problem is my wife. She really needs to change the way she talks to me

Patient Statement #6 I don't like using forms, and surveys. They are too technical.

Patient Statement #7 First I need to sleep better, then I can quit smoking pot.

Patient Statement #8 I'm not the type that does homework

Patient Statement #9 First, I need to get over this depression, then I'll feel that life is worth living and won't contemplate suicide.

For these next statements, the patient is challenging and reluctant to get to work.

Patient Statement #10 I can't keep going with this depression and feeling so hopeless. Nothing is going to work.

Patient Statement #11 The real problem isn't my drinking; it's just that I'm depressed. I could quit anytime, and I'm just self-medicating the depression.

Patient Statement #12 I am the one doing all the work in this relationship, but I am not ready to give up on her yet. She just needs to change the way she talks to me.

Trainees should attempt to improvise their own responses before reading the example responses (Table 12.2).

Table 12.2 Example therapist responses: gentle ultimatum

	Patient statement	Example therapist response
Patient statement #1	I am tired of feeling this much anxiety and need to get some relief from it.	The only way I know to cure anxiety is with a heavy dose of exposure work that is outside of your comfort zone. (Criteria 1 and 3) I'd be delighted to do this with you. (Criterion 4) It's very rewarding but it is hard. (Criterion 2) However, I would totally understand if it's not something you'd be willing to do to overcome your anxiety. (Criterion 5)
Patient statement #2	I want to figure out the communication in my relationship, but my partner doesn't ever listen.	This is a real dilemma because I don't know how to help anyone transform the communication in their relationship (Criterion 3) unless they are 100% willing to look at their role. (Criterion 1) It would be a pleasure to work with you and the potential is good (Criterion 4), but it will take a ton of effort and be very humbling. (Criterion 2) I completely understand if you don't want to sign up for this approach. (Criterion 5)
Patient statement #3	I have tried everything to manage my anxiety, nothing seems to last.	The way I know to cure anxiety is with exposure work that is done right. (Criteria 1 and 3) It's very rewarding, but it is very hard (Criterion 2). I'd be delighted to do this with you. (Criterion 4) And would also totally understand if it's not something you'd be willing to do (Criterion 5).

(continued)

Table 12.2 (continued)

	Patient statement	Example therapist response
Patient statement #4	I just can't seem to get around to doing my taxes.	There are two key things that will be required to get that goal you have of doing your taxes. The first is that you will need to commit to a scheduled time and sit down at your desk and get started even when you don't feel like it. The second is that you will have to set up accountability with someone to let them know you completed it (Criterion 1). Now I would love to work with you to set this up, (Criterion 4) but I don't know how to help anyone get their paperwork completed without these conditions. (Criterion 3) I realize this will not be easy. (Criterion 2) I fully understand if you are hesitant to move forward with this plan and leave the decision 100% up to you. (Criterion 5)
Patient statement #5	The problem is my wife. She really needs to change the way she talks to me.	I'm not sure if I can help you with that because the only way I know how to help people with their relationship is if they assume 100% responsibility for the problems in the relationship. (Criteria 1 and 3) It's not fair because a relationship is a two-way street, and your wife is clearly being very hurtful and here we are asking you to assume all the blame anyway. It also requires a lot of hard work on your part to examine your role, revise your communication, and respond to her with zero blame even when she's being very unreasonable. (Criteria 1, 2) I love relationship work and will be with you every step of the way, (Criterion 4) but completely understand if that's not something you'd be willing to do. (Criterion 5)
Patient statement #6	I don't like using forms and surveys. They are too technical.	Forms are technical and take some time and effort to complete. (Criterion 2) I want to make sure I am clear on how we can be effective because it would be wonderful to work together with you. (Criterion 4) The challenge is that I don't know how to help people without using the forms before and after every session. (Criterion 3) That may seem like a big request when you don't like filling out forms. (Criterion 2) I am optimistic that we can get the result you are looking for (Criterion 4) but I wouldn't want to pressure you in any way if you don't think that this approach is for you. (Criterion 5)
Patient statement #7	First, I need to sleep better, then I can quit smoking pot.	It makes sense. The problem is that I don't know how to help people overcome sleep problems while they continue to use marijuana. (Criterion 3) Don't get me wrong, I have nothing against Marijuana. It is not a moral issue. It's just that getting high and also withdrawals from marijuana both would shortcircuit our efforts to help your body learn to sleep without marijuana. This means that in order to sleep better and overcome that problem completely you'd have to first stop smoking, for a long time before your sleep will improve. (Criteria 1 and 2) I'd be happy to do this with you (Criterion 4) but also completely understand if it's just not worth it to you to quit smoking only to improve sleep. (Criterion 5)

(continued)

Table 12.2 (continued)

	Patient statement	Example therapist response
Patient statement #8	I'm not the type that does homework.	Homework is hard, especially if you're not the type who does it. (Criterion 2) While I would really love to work with you, I have to admit that I don't know how to help anyone without assigning daily homework. (Criteria 3 and 4) That may sound pretty demanding, and it is. (Criterion 2) Perhaps this type of therapy that requires homework isn't the style you could commit to and that is completely understandable. I would be sad to see you go, as I think it could be fun to work with others, but I fully support you if you choose to work with someone who does not require homework. (Criterion 5)
Patient statement #9	First, I need to get over this depression, then I'll feel that life is worth living and won't contemplate suicide.	I can see the logic in what you're saying, but at the same time, I don't know how to help people overcome depression as long as suicide is on the table. (Criterion 3) In order to overcome depression, you'd need to first give up, for good, on the idea that you could end your life. (Criterion 1) It's hard to do, and often the thought of being able to end your life can serve as a respite from the hardships of life. Taking away your ability to end your own life can also feel like something that is yours and your right is taken away from you. (Criterion 2) All of that is completely understandable and will require some hard work together to find out if you'd be willing to put suicide off the table for the rest of your life, (Criteria 1, 2, and 4) but I also completely understand if that means asking too much of you just so you could have a chance of overcoming depression and that it may not be worth it to you. (Criterion 5)
Patient statement #10	I can't keep going with this depression and feeling so hopeless. Nothing is going to work.	It may sound unrealistic for you to hear that the potential for recovery is very good because depression is super challenging and can feel hopeless. But you deserve to know what it is I can offer you and what you will have to do to recover. (Criterion 2) The reality is that I don't know how to help you with your depression and hopelessness without a couple of critical tasks. (Criterion 3) The first is that you and I will have to focus on and work hard in our sessions to discover the tools and strategies that will work for you; the second is that you will have to do daily homework for 20–30 minutes a day even when you don't feel like it. (Criterion 1) I would love to work with you to help you overcome this depression, (Criterion 4) at the same time, it is entirely your decision if you want to sign up for this kind of therapy or if you choose this isn't for you. (Criterion 5)

(continued)

Table 12.2 (continued)

	Patient statement	Example therapist response
Patient statement #11	The real problem isn't my drinking; it's just that I'm depressed. I could quit anytime, and I'm just self-medicating the depression.	Absolutely. The real problem is depression. However, I don't know how to help people overcome depression as long as they drink. (Criterion 3) This could feel very unfair, as I'm sure alcohol is one of the few breaks you get. And now don't get me wrong, I have nothing against alcohol, it's not a moral issue, it's just that I don't know how to help you learn to negotiate life's difficulties and depression while your brain is affected by alcohol use or when it's withdrawing. (Criterion 3) To overcome depression, unfortunately, you'd need to first get completely sober for a long time (Criterion 1) and that won't be easy. (Criterion 2) I'd be happy to help you in every step of the way and do whatever it takes to overcome your depression. (Criterion 4) At the same time, I wouldn't fault you at all if you decided that the price to pay is too high and that you're not ready to tackle it at this time. (Criterion 5)
Patient statement #12	I am the one doing all the work in this relationship, but I am not ready to give up on her yet. She just needs to change the way she talks to me.	It would be a tremendous pleasure to work with you to turn your relationship around and get that closeness and connection with your wife that you desire (Criterion 4). But before we jump in, you deserve to know what that will take, as it is no small task. (Criterion 2) This may seem very unfair, but I don't know how to help people with relationship difficulties without these three components. One, we will be focusing 100% on your role and seeing what it is you can do to change. Two, you will have to be willing to give up blaming your wife for the problems. Three, I will be asking you to do daily writing homework where you analyze how you are interacting with her and look at all the errors, you're making so you can practice new ways to communicate. (Criterion 1) That may sound like a lot, and it is a big ask considering how much you are already doing in the relationship. (Criterion 2) I don't want to pressure you in any way and fully support you if you decide that now is not the right time to work on it. (Criterion 5)

Chapter 13
Capturing and Refining Negative Thoughts

Skill Description

The hallmark of the cognitive part of CBT is helping patients untwist their distorted negative thoughts, which in turn impacts how they feel. "Negative thoughts" are any thoughts that cause unnecessary stress or pain.[1] The first step is to capture the patient's negative thoughts. This is an uncovering technique, so the therapist and patient become more aware of the patient's inner experience. It also prepares the therapist and patient to confront the negative thoughts later. In the process, we also listen and provide empathy for the patient's experience, thereby strengthening the therapeutic relationship.

In TEAM-CBT, we aim to capture negative thoughts while resisting the urge to prematurely "help" our patient. Offering help prematurely, before adequately empathizing, can evoke the patient's resistance to conscience awareness and melt it away. Therefore, as we capture the patient's negative thoughts, we need to resist the urge to bring attention to the thoughts as distorted or negative. The goal is to non-judgmentally gather data, become aware of the thoughts, and write them down.

Keep a writing pad ready, and continuously keep an eye out and hunt for negative thoughts, especially during the following times:

1. Earlier in the therapy hour, while we mainly connect and empathize with our patient, we can note negative thoughts. We do this without pointing them out. The therapist takes note of the thoughts, verbatim, with a plan for them to be used later.

---

[1] If the thought does not cause unnecessary pain or stress, then it is not a negative thought. For example, I could be depressed and say to myself "I'll never amount to anything," which would make me feel worse. However I could also say "I'll never amount to anything" without it causing pain or distress, rather with acceptance and relief. See Chap. 10 for use of the Acceptance Paradox.

© The Author(s), under exclusive license to Springer Nature Switzerland AG 2023
M. Katz et al., *Deliberate Practice of TEAM-CBT*, SpringerBriefs in Psychology,
https://doi.org/10.1007/978-3-031-46019-7_13

2. During the Specificity step in Agenda Setting (Chap. 7), while there is an upsetting event and the patient is expressing the emotions they were feeling at that moment, we can ask the patient what they were thinking or saying to themself as they were experiencing it. We can also tie thoughts to emotions by asking questions such as "I hear you were feeling anxious. What were some of your anxious thoughts?"

3. After we have dealt with Outcome and Process Resistance (Chaps. 9, 10, 11 & 12), and we are finally ready to use the many Cognitive and Behavioral methods, TEAM-CBT has to offer as part of the Methods section of the therapy work, we flush out in writing the negative thoughts we will soon be confronting.

In this exercise, you will practice distilling the patients' negative thoughts and writing them down using the following rules: convert questions into statements, look for hidden "should statements" and make them explicit, and divide the patient's statements into as many negative thoughts as possible.

Examples of This Skill in Practice

Example #1

Patient: I'm lying in bed last night, my wife was next to me, and all I was thinking was that I feel so hopeless! Why am I so depressed? I mean, when will I ever get better?

Therapist: Absolutely, you were feeling hopeless and telling yourself "I should be better by now" (Criterion 2) and "I shouldn't be so hopeless" (Criterion 2) and I hear other hopeless thoughts in there such as "I will never get better." (Criterion 1) Let's write these down. (Criterion 3)

Example #2

Patient: I am so frustrated with myself. I got so anxious last weekend when I had to meet my girlfriend's parents and I am sure they were disappointed. What is wrong with me?

Therapist: Absolutely! Let's write these down as three negative thoughts (Criterion 3):

1. I shouldn't have gotten so anxious last weekend. (Criterion 2)
2. My girlfriend's parents are definitely disappointed in me. (Criterion 1)
3. There must be something wrong with me. (Criterion 1)

Example #3

Patient: In my head, I kept wondering, "What if I have another panic attack?" I feel so anxious weeks before, when I have to travel, but I can't possibly go on another flight! My family is going to be so disappointed that we can't go on the family vacation!

Therapist: It sounds like that question is coming from the idea or thought: "I am going to have another panic attack." (Criterion 1) Let's write that down as thought

#1. (Criterion 3) I'm hearing a couple of other negative thoughts too, such as (Criterion 1): "I can't go on another flight," "I'll disappoint my family," "we won't be able to go on a family vacation," and also "I shouldn't feel so anxious." (Criterion 2) Can we write these down as well? (Criterion 3)

Now it is your turn: Follow the Exercise Instructions and Skill Criteria Table 13.1).

After 15 minutes of practice, the patient and therapist switch roles and start over.

These next statements include patient statements that are mildly challenging to refine and consolidate into negative thoughts.

Patient Statement #1 I can't seem to get out of this feeling of depression and that I won't get better. Why am I like this? I am such a loser.

Patient Statement #2 I can't go back to class. Whenever I set foot in there, I can already tell nobody likes me, everybody is talking among themselves and seems much happier to see each other than they are to see me. If we have to divide into groups, nobody will want to be with me. I guess I have to accept that nobody likes me. I'm just unloveable.

Patient Statement #3 I am so worried that my partner is going to leave me. She says that I am too anxious and need to relax, but I feel stressed all the time. What will I do if she leaves? My life will be a mess. Why can't I get a handle on this?

Table 13.1 Criteria for capturing and refining negative thoughts practice exercise

---

The therapist improvises a response to each patient statement using the following criteria:
   1. Break down the patients' statements and questions into as many negative thoughts as possible.
   2. Uncover implicit "should" statements and make them explicit.
   3. Ask the patient to write it (the negative thought) down (both the therapist and the patient write it down).
Proceed to the next patient statement only when it is too easy for the therapist to meet all criteria.

Patient Statement #4 I know I'm supposed to be productive and work on some of the assignments my manager asked me to do, but I feel so annoyed that I have to do this super tedious work that nobody will actually look at, and then my mom is on my case! I mean, why does she need to try to manage my life? I just want to give myself a break and play a little chess online or watch some TikTok videos and before I know it, it's already 5 AM.

> ***These next statements include patient statements that are moderately challenging to refine and consolidate into negative thoughts.***

Patient Statement #5 I am such a fraud at work. I don't really know what I am doing. What if my boss discovers that I am just putting in time? Everyone else is better than me, and I am sure they all think I am the weak link on the team. How long can I keep this up before they fire me?

Patient Statement #6 Relationship OCD: I get really worried that maybe I've lost all of my passion for my girlfriend, that maybe I don't actually love her and she isn't the one, I mean how can I tell? What if my passion never comes back?

Patient Statement #7 Who knows what is going to happen with the economy these days? I am already maxed out with my budget, and everything keeps getting more expensive. What if we can't sell our house? How will I ever get out of this pressure? I feel so overwhelmed. What is the point of all this hard work anyway?

Patient Statement #8 I lay in bed at night, and that's when it grips me; one day the world will end and it will be the end of all of life and humanity, there will be nothing! I feel so much fear, and it's so silly, I've had these fears since I was eight years old! And the problem is there's no answer to these fears because it's true! So I'm destined to always feel these fears, probably more and more as I get older myself!

> ***These next statements include patient statements that are challenging to refine and consolidate into negative thoughts.***

Patient Statement #9 I mean, what's the point? Once trust is lost, it's very hard to regain, and since I hid and lied about failing at my school, my father will never trust me again. They will always see me as a corrupt person, and I can't blame them, I am a corrupt person.

Patient Statement #10 I don't know how I will survive without my husband. What am I going to do? What if I am all alone? Where will I live? I don't want to be a burden to the kids, but I have never taken care of the finances. I am so scared he will never recover, and I will lose him.

Patient Statement #11 We go to the cabin with the family, and everybody drinks around me, and I know it would taste so good and be so relaxing to have a few, and it's so unfair that everybody else gets to enjoy themselves and I don't. And what's really annoying is that my wife doesn't even care that I'm struggling. She just gives me a hard time that I don't want to hang out with everyone because they are drinking and being stupid together.

Patient Statement #12 No matter what I do, I always feel so overwhelmed. It is never-ending with the constant expectations of kids, work, and my marriage. There isn't enough time in the day and my list keeps getting longer. I never get any space for myself. Why am I like this? When will it ever end?

Trainees should attempt to improvise their own responses before reading the example responses (Table 13.2)

Table 13.2 Example therapist responses: capturing and refining negative thoughts

	Patient statement	Example therapist response
Patient statement #1	I can't seem to get of under this feeling of depression and that I won't get better. Why am I like this? I am such a loser.	I'm hearing some hidden should statements in there, like "I should be better by now" and "I shouldn't be this depressed." (Criterion 1 and 2) Do you see that too? I'm also hearing the negative thought "I'm a loser" (Criterion 1) let's write those three down. (Criterion 3)
Patient statement #2	I can't go back to class. Whenever I set foot in there, I can already tell nobody likes me, everybody is talking among themselves and seems much happier to see each other than they are to see me. If we have to divide into groups, nobody will want to be with me. I guess I have to accept that nobody likes me. I'm just unloveable.	It sounds like you are having a number of negative thoughts when you feel anxious. Let's capture those and write them down. (Criterion 3) I heard you say: "I can't go back to class." "Nobody likes me." "Everybody is happier to see each other than they are to see me." "Nobody will want to be with me if we divide into groups" and "I am just unlovable." (Criterion 1)
Patient statement #3	I am so worried that my partner is going to leave me. She says that I am too anxious and need to relax, but I feel stressed all the time. What will I do if she leaves? My life will be a mess. Why can't I get a handle on this?	Let's capture the negative thoughts in your statement, find should statements, and convert questions into statements. I'm hearing these: 1. I'm stressed all the time. 2. I won't make it if she leaves. (Criterion 1) 3. If she leaves, my life will be a mess. (Criterion 1) 4. I should be able to get a handle on this (Criteria 2) Can you see that? Let's write them down. (Criterion 3)

(continued)

Table 13.2 (continued)

	Patient statement	Example therapist response
Patient statement #4	I know I'm supposed to be productive and work on some of the assignments my manager asked me to do, but I feel so annoyed that I have to do this super tedious work that nobody will actually look at, and then my mom is on my case! I mean, why does she need to try to manage my life? I just want to give myself a break and play a little chess online or watch some TikTok videos and before I know it, it's already 5 AM	There seem to be a few negative thoughts that I am hearing from you. Let's list them together (Criterion 3): 1. I should be more productive at work. (Criterion 2) 2. I shouldn't have to do tedious work. (Criterion 2) 3. No one will look at or appreciate the work I do. (Criterion 1) 4. My mom shouldn't be on my case and try to manage my life. (Criteria 1)
Patient statement #5	I am such a fraud at work. I don't really know what I am doing. What if my boss discovers that I am just putting in time? Everyone else is better than me and I am sure they all think I am the weak link on the team. How long can I keep this up before they fire me?	Let's find the negative thoughts in your statements and write them down: (Criterion 3) I'm hearing: 1. I'm a fraud at work. (Criteria 1) 2. I don't know what I'm doing. (Criteria 1) 3. I should be better than this. (Criterion 2) 4. My boss will discover that I'm just putting in time and that will be horrible. (Criteria 1) 5. Everyone else is better than me. (Criteria 1) 6. They all think I'm the weak link. (Criteria 1) 7. They are going to fire me. (Criteria 1)
Patient statement #6	I get really worried that maybe I've lost all of my passion for my girlfriend, that maybe I don't actually love her and she isn't the one, I mean how can I tell? What if my passion never comes back?	Let's capture some of those negative thoughts you have when you feel anxious. It sounds like you are telling yourself: 1. I have lost my passion for my girlfriend. (Criterion 1) 2. I should know if I love her. (Criterion 2) 3. I should know if she is the one. (Criterion 2) 4. My passion will never come back if I lose it. (Criterion 1) Let's write those down together. (Criterion 3)
Patient statement #7	Who knows what is going to happen with the economy these days? I am already maxed out with my budget and everything keeps getting more expensive. What if we can't sell our house? How will I ever get out of this pressure? I feel so overwhelmed. What is the point of all this hard work anyway?	Let's write down the negative thoughts hidden within your words: (Criteria 3) 1. We won't be able to sell our house. (Criterion 1) 2. I will never get out of this pressure. (Criterion 1) 3. I shouldn't feel so overwhelmed. (Criterion 2) 4. There's no point to all this. (Criterion 1)

(continued)

Table 13.2 (continued)

	Patient statement	Example therapist response
Patient statement #8	I lay in bed at night and that's when it grips me, one day the world will end and it will be the end of all of life and humanity, there will be nothing! I feel so much fear, and it's so silly, I've had these fears since I was eight years old! And the problem is there's no answer to these fears because it's true! So I'm destined to always feel these fears, probably more and more as I get older myself!	It sounds like there are a number of negative thoughts that are coming up for you. Here are the ones that I noticed: 1. One day, the world, life, and humanity will end. (Criterion 1) 2. There will be nothing. (Criterion 1) 3. I shouldn't be so silly. (Criterion 2) 4. There is no answer to these fears. (Criterion 1) 5. I will never overcome these fears. (Criterion 1) 6. It will get worse as I get older. (Criterion 1) Let's write those down. (Criterion 3)
Patient statement #9	I mean, what's the point? Once trust is lost, it's very hard to regain, and since I hid and lied about failing at my school, my father will never trust me again. They will always see me as a corrupt person and I can't blame them, I am a corrupt person.	I'm hearing a number of negative thoughts in your statements. Here's what I'm hearing: 1. There's no point. (Criterion 1) 2. There should be a point. (Criterion 2) 3. My father will never trust me again. (Criterion 1) 4. They will always see me as a corrupt person. (Criterion 1) 5. They should always see me as a corrupt person. (Criterion 2) 6. I am a corrupt person. (Criterion 1) Let's write all of these down. (Criterion 3)
Patient statement #10	I don't know how I will survive without my husband. What am I going to do? What if I am all alone? Where will I live? I don't want to be a burden to the kids, but I have never taken care of the finances. I am so scared he will never recover, and I will lose him.	You mentioned a number of things that you are thinking about. Let's write them down as negative thoughts (Criterion 3) Here is what I heard you say: 1. I won't survive without my husband. (Criterion 1) 2. I won't know what to do. (Criterion 1) 3. I will be all alone. (Criterion 1) 4. I don't have anywhere to live. (Criterion 1). 5. I will be a burden to my kids. (Criterion 1) 6. I won't be able to take care of the finances. (Criterion 1) 7. My husband will never recover. (Criterion 1) 8. I will lose him. (Criterion 1)

(continued)

Table 13.2 (continued)

	Patient statement	Example therapist response
Patient statement #11	We go to the cabin with the family and everybody drinks around me, and I know it would taste so good and be so relaxing to have a few, and it's so unfair that everybody else gets to enjoy themselves and I don't. Can't they even see that they have a problem with alcohol? And what's really annoying is that my wife doesn't even care that I'm struggling. She just gives me a hard time that I don't want to hang out with everyone because they are drinking and being stupid together.	Let's capture some of the negative thoughts you're saying: 1. It's not fair that I don't get to drink. (Criterion 1) 2. I should be allowed to drink. (Criterion 2) 3. My wife doesn't care that I'm struggling. (Criteria 1) 4. They should be able to see they have a problem with alcohol. (Criteria 2) 5. My wife shouldn't give me such a hard time. (Criterion 2) 6. They shouldn't be doing this. (Criterion 2) 7. They are just being stupid. 8. It won't be enjoyable unless I drink. (Criterion 1) Let's write all of these down as negative thoughts. (Criterion 3)
Patient statement #12	No matter what I do, I always feel so overwhelmed. It is never-ending with the constant expectations of kids, work, and my marriage. There isn't enough time in the day and my list keeps getting longer. I never get any space for myself. Why am I like this? When will it ever end?	Ugh, so hard! Here are the negative thoughts that I'm hearing you say: 1. I shouldn't feel so overwhelmed. (Criterion 2) 2. The hard work is constant. 3. The hard work is never-ending. 4. I never do enough. 5. I should be able to do more. (Criterion 2) 6. I never get any space for myself. 7. It shouldn't be like this. (Criterion 2) 8. Things will never get better. (Criterion 1) Can you write them down with me? (Criterion 3)

Chapter 14
Cognitive Role-Playing Techniques: Externalization of Voices

Skill Description

Cognitive Role-Playing techniques are one of the hallmarks of TEAM-CBT. They are often the highlight of our sessions and provide some of the most memorable and meaningful breakthrough moments for our patients. However, they should not be used before we are convinced that the patient has brought all of the good reasons not to change into their conscious awareness, and has melted away the resistance to change by using the five steps of Agenda Setting (see Chaps. 6–12). If used too early, they carry a high risk of falling flat. To perform them well, the therapist will need a list of the patient's negative thoughts written verbatim, preferably with a measure from 0 to 100% of how much the patient believes each of their negative thoughts to be true. (Table 14.1)

Our goal is to confront our patients with their negative thoughts and have them experience responding to them verbally, out loud, *with thought through arguments*, instead of silently inside their heads.

In all cognitive role-play techniques, the therapist will always take the role of the negative thought first, in order to put the patient in a position to confront their own negative thoughts and overcome them themselves using their own arguments and reason. A common and unfortunate mistake we see is when the patient takes on the role of the negative thought in the cognitive role-play, leaving the therapist to try and convince them that their negative thoughts are not true, which can encourage the patient to dig their heels in.

Only if we feel that the patient is having a hard time responding effectively to their negative thoughts do we reverse roles. We do so briefly, give them some suggestions as to how to defeat that negative thought while we are in the role of the positive. We then quickly reverse once more, so the therapist can be back in the role of the negative thought again. We urge you to never feel comfortable taking the voice of positive responses to your patients' negative thoughts.

© The Author(s), under exclusive license to Springer Nature Switzerland AG 2023   95
M. Katz et al., *Deliberate Practice of TEAM-CBT*, SpringerBriefs in Psychology,
https://doi.org/10.1007/978-3-031-46019-7_14

Table 14.1 Example of negative thoughts and measurement

Negative thoughts	% Belief before	% Belief after
Everybody hates me	80%	
Nobody likes me in my school	75%	
I'm unlovable	75%	
I don't have any friends	50%	

When you first start practicing the technique, you may find it intimidating or cruel to "attack" your patients with these negative statements. After all, what kind of therapist wants to say to their patient that they are unlovable? Remember, it is not that the therapist is cruel, it is that the patient's self-talk is cruel, and you are helping them overcome it.

Once your patient starts winning against their negative thought, you can abandon, at least for the moment, the confrontational negative thought and use Thought Empathy (Repeating in agreement what they said verbatim, see Exercise 2) to help them build their argument against the negative thought. Then, once their argument seems more and more successful, you can go back to the voice of the negative thought and "hit" them with it again, so to give the patient another chance to respond to it.

There are several cognitive role-playing techniques in TEAM-CBT: Externalization of Voices, Devil's Advocate, Feared Fantasy Technique, the Double Standard Technique, to name a few. Once you get the spirit of one, you will find the rest are very easy to learn. They all follow the same pattern:

1. Introduction/setup: Describe the technique to the patient.
2. Delivery: Attack the patient with their negative thoughts as they confront them one by one.
3. Processing: Ask the patient to write down their winning arguments against the negative thoughts.

Examples of This Skill in Practice

Example #1
Patient's negative thought: I'm no good.
Therapist statement: I'm going to role-play the negative voice in your head. Your job is to defeat me. (Criterion 1) Are you ready? (Criterion 2) Joe, can I speak with you? I'd like to remind you that "You are no good!" (Criterion 3)

Example #2
Patient's negative thought: I'm never going to amount to anything.
Therapist statement: I am going to be the negative voice in your head, and your role is to argue back and try to defeat me (Criterion 1). Are you ready? (Criterion

2) "Hi Billy, I'm that voice in your head and wanted to let you know that "You're never going to amount to anything!" (Criterion 3).

Example #3

Patient's negative thought: Nobody likes me at work.

Therapist: How about I'll be the negative voice in your head, and your job will be to defeat me. (Criterion 1) Ready to be attacked by your negative thoughts? (Criterion 2) "OK I'm the voice of your negative thoughts and I need to tell you the truth, "Nobody likes you at work!" (Criterion 3)

Now it's your turn: Follow the Exercise Instructions and Skill Criteria (Table 14.2).

After 15 minutes of practice, the patient and therapist switch roles and start over.

Patient's Negative Thought #1 Nothing will ever change.

Patient's Negative Thought #2 I have failed at everything in life.

Patient's Negative Thought #3 No one understands me.

Patient's Negative Thought #4 I won't be able to cope without my husband.

Patient's Negative Thought #5 It's all my fault that my dad left.

Patient's Negative Thought #6 I am going to freeze and make a fool of myself in this interview.

Table 14.2 Criteria for externalization of voices practice exercise

The therapist improvises a response to each patient statement using the following criteria:
1. State that you are going to take on the role of their negative voice and their job is to defeat you.
2. Ask if the patient is ready to start the role-play.
3. Attack the patient with their negative thoughts using the second person, "You" (verbatim with no other changes or alterations).
Proceed to the next patient statement only when it is too easy for the therapist to meet all criteria.

Patient's Negative Thought #7 Everyone is judging me because I made a mistake at work.

Patient's Negative Thought #8 I need to be close to someone to truly be happy.

Patient's Negative Thought #9 I will never get out of this rut.

Patient's Negative Thought #10 I am a complete loser.

Patient's Negative Thought #11 I will be all alone if something happens to my brother.

Patient's Negative Thought #12 Nobody likes me.

Trainees should attempt to improvise their own responses before reading the example responses (Table 14.3)

Table 14.3 Example therapist responses: externalization of voices

	Patient statement	Example therapist response
Patient's negative thought #1	Nothing will ever change.	I am going to be you and play your negative voice and you try to defeat me. (Criteria 1 and 2) Ready? (Criterion 2) I just wanted to let you know that "Nothing will ever change." (Criterion 3)
Patient's negative thought #2	I have failed at everything in life.	OK, now I'll play your negative thought, and you try to defeat me. (Criterion 1) Ready? (Criterion 2) "You've failed at everything in life!" (Criterion 3)
Patient's negative thought #3	No one understands me.	In this role-play, you will be your positive voice, and I will play the role of your negative thoughts. Your job is to defeat me. (Criterion 1) Here we go, are you ready? (Criterion 2) "No one understands you." (Criterion 3)
Patient's negative thought #4	I won't be able to cope without my husband.	Now, I'll take on the voice of your negative thoughts and you try to defeat me. (Criterion 1) Are you ready? (Criterion 2) "You won't be able to cope without your husband!" (Criterion 3)
Patient's negative thought #5	It's all my fault that my dad left.	I am going to be your negative voice in this role-play, and your job is to argue back against me while playing the positive voice. (Criterion 1) Let's get started, are you ready? (Criterion 2) "It's all your fault that your dad left." (Criterion 3)
Patient's negative thought #6	I am going to freeze and make a fool of myself in this interview.	I'll pretend to be your negative thoughts, and your job will be to stand up to me. (Criterion 1) Ready? (Criterion 2) Listen, "You're going to freeze and make a fool of yourself in this interview!" (Criterion 3)
Patient's negative thought #7	Everyone is judging me because I made a mistake at work.	In this role-play, you will be the positive, rational, and reasonable self, and I will play the role of your negative thoughts. Your job is to defeat me. (Criterion 1) Ready? (Criterion 2) "Everyone is judging you because you made a mistake at work." (Criterion 3)

(continued)

Table 14.3 (continued)

	Patient statement	Example therapist response
Patient's negative thought #8	I need to be close to someone to truly be happy.	How about I be the voice of your negative thoughts and you try to defeat me? (Criterion 1) Here we go, are you ready? (Criterion 2) Listen! "the only way you could be happy is to be close to someone", there's no other way. (Criterion 3)
Patient's negative thought #9	I will never get out of this rut.	Let's jump into this role-play where you will be positive "you" and I will be negative "you." You convince me that you are right and I am wrong about this thought. (Criterion 1) All set? (Criterion 2) "You will never get out of this rut." (Criterion 3)
Patient's negative thought #10	I am a complete loser.	OK, now can we role-play where I take on the voice of your negative thoughts and your job is to defeat me? (Criterion 1) Here we go, are you ready? (Criterion 2) Listen John, "You are a complete loser!" (Criterion 3)
Patient's negative thought #11	I will be all alone if something happens to my brother.	This is a powerful role-play technique where I will be you, but I am going to be the negative you and you will be the positive. Your job is to crush me by arguing back and convincing me that I am wrong. (Criterion 1) Ready? (Criterion 2) "You will be all alone if something happens to your brother." (Criterion 3)
Patient's negative thought #12	Nobody likes me.	Let's use a technique where I take on the role of your negative thoughts and your job is to respond to me, (Criterion 1) Ready? (Criterion 2) Listen Maya, the truth is that "nobody likes you!" (Criterion 3)

Chapter 15
Helping Patients Understand How to Defeat Their Negative Thoughts

Skill Description

In this skill, you will practice teaching patients how they can talk back to their negative thoughts in an effective way during role-play. In TEAM-CBT, therapists use a wide variety of cognitive role-play techniques (see Chap. 14). Throughout all role-plays, it is important to teach patients skills that they can use first with us, and then without us to defeat their negative thoughts. In this technique, patients are taught three kinds of approaches. A good response can involve all three:

1. *Acceptance paradox*: Accepting the truth in the negative thought paradoxically deflates it. For example, an acceptance paradox response to "I am a failure" could be: "That's 100% true! I have failed in so many things in my life, and plan to continue to learn and grow and fail in many things in the future. I wouldn't want it any other way, because if I didn't fail, I wouldn't learn anything. I can take the pressure off, relax and enjoy my little life failing and learning along the way."
2. *Self-defense*: Use logic and reason to poke holes at the negative thought. For example, if the negative thought is "I am a failure," a self-defense response would poke holes at the negative thought by saying things such as "I'm not a failure, I'm just human and there are some things I have succeeded in like school, friendships, and being there for people who need me."
3. *Counterattack*: Talk back to the negative voice itself rather than to the content of what it is saying. For example, to the thought "I am a failure" one could say, "Yeah yeah, I know you cruel depressive voice, I'm not listening to you anymore!" or "Oh here's that thought again, that I'm a failure, I'm not going to let you bother me anymore."

It is often said that if defeating negative thoughts would be a boxing match, any win is a great win. However, winning with the self-defense technique is similar to

M. Katz et al., *Deliberate Practice of TEAM-CBT*, SpringerBriefs in Psychology, https://doi.org/10.1007/978-3-031-46019-7_15

winning the match by points, while winning with the acceptance paradox is more like winning by knockout.

Sometimes it is useful for the therapist to model the skills, and even make it personal to them. We encourage you to use self-disclosure and give an example related to a personal negative thought you have struggled with to enhance the therapeutic alliance and make it authentic.

Patients are usually taught these skills through an iterative process while simultaneously engaging in cognitive role-play. When working with your patient, therapists should notice which of the three approaches they get and which ones they miss. Then, the therapist can reverse roles and use the ones that the patient did not use. Remember, we only suggest ways to defeat your patients' negative thoughts in order to stimulate their own thinking, so they can put it in their own words and process it themselves. Therefore, right after the patient hears from you how to defeat their thoughts, the roles should be quickly reversed again, so the patient takes back the role of defeating their own negative thoughts. Therapists can reverse the roles by saying something like "I see you agree with what I'm saying against this thought, great! Now can you say it in your own words?"

This exercise was intentionally designed so you, as the therapist, could learn how to respond to some of the more common negative thoughts people have.

The exercise is structured to be progressively harder by asking you to use more of the three strategies with each thought.

Examples of This Skill in Practice

Context: All patient statements occur after the patient has tried unsuccessfully to respond to a negative thought in the context of role-play.

Example #1 – For Criterion 2, Only Use Acceptance Paradox
Patient: I am just not sure how to defeat this thought, "I am no good."
Therapist: I can sense you're a little stuck here. Here is one way you might consider: (Criterion 1) "It is a huge relief that I am no good. I used to have all this pressure to be successful. Now I realize that I am just human with flaws and failures and this unrealistic expectation was just causing me pain. Now I am free, thanks for reminding me that I am no good." (Criterion 2a) (*short pause*) How about you try and put it into your own words? (Criterion 3)

Example #2 – For Criterion 2, Use Self-defense and Acceptance Paradox
Patient: I am stuck on this thought, "I'm never going to amount to anything."
Therapist: Yeah, I sense you're a little stuck, how about I try and respond to it? (Criterion 1) "It's true that I haven't lived up to my full potential, absolutely, and I had hoped to be more accomplished by now, and that's OK, I will continue to strive and work to improve myself, maybe for the rest of my life. (Criterion 2a) At the same time, I've already amounted to something! I have friends who care about me and I care about them. I graduated from college, and I accomplish

many small things each and every day." (Criterion 2b) (Pause) Does any of this resonate with you? Can you try to answer back to this negative thought now?" (Criterion 3)

Example #3 – For Criterion 2, Use Self-defense, Acceptance Paradox, And Counterattack

Patient: I don't know how to respond to this thought; it seems true, "Nobody likes me at work."

Therapist: It sounds like you are a little stuck with this one. How about I try to model some responses? (Criterion 1) "Just because my boss is critical does not mean that no one likes me. My coworkers agree that he can be harsh and they interact with me. (Criterion 2b) Truthfully, it would be a pain if everyone at work liked me and was constantly wanting to chat and hang out. I like my space. It is a good thing that some people don't like me. Sometimes I don't like myself so they can just join the crowd. (Criterion 2a) The real problem is that I keep listening to that negative self talk you keep bringing up. So just stop it." (Criterion 2c) (Pause). Now you try the parts that worked for you and put them into your words. (Criterion 3)

Now it is your turn: Follow the Exercise Instructions and Skill Criteria (Table 15.1).

After 15 minutes of practice, the patient and therapist switch roles and start over.

Context: All patient statements occur during the patient trying unsuccessfully to respond to their negative thoughts in the context of cognitive role-play.

Patient Statement #1 I can't seem to figure out how to challenge this thought, "Nothing will ever change."

Table 15.1 Criteria for defeating negative thoughts practice exercise

The therapist improvises a response to each patient statement using the following criteria:
  1. Acknowledge that the patient is feeling stuck and suggest that you model some options for them to try.
  2. The therapist models a response using one or more of these strategies:
      (a) Acceptance paradox
      (b) Self-defense
      (c) Counterattack
  3. After a short pause, ask the patient to try it in their own words.
Proceed to the next patient statement only when it is too easy for the therapist to meet all criteria.

> *For these next statements, in order to meet Criterion 2, the therapist has to only use ACCEPTANCE PARADOX.*

Patient Statement #2 This idea has me stuck: "I have failed at everything in life."

Patient Statement #3 I just can't see how to defeat this thought, "No one understands me."

Patient Statement #4 I am stuck on this one: "I won't be able to cope without my husband."

> *For these next statements, in order to meet Criterion 2, the therapist has to use ACCEPTANCE PARADOX and SELF-DEFENSE.*

Patient Statement #5 I am not sure how to respond to this idea: "It's all my fault that my dad left."

Patient Statement #6 This one is just true; I can't answer that "I am going to freeze and make a fool of myself in this interview."

Patient Statement #7 I am stuck on how to respond to the thought, "Everyone is judging me because I made a mistake at work."

Patient Statement #8 This is hard, I don't know how to answer that "I need to be close to someone to truly be happy."

Patient Statement #9 This one is so hard for me to challenge: "I will never get out of this rut."

Patient Statement #10 Here is the one that I get tripped up by: "I am a complete loser."

> *For these next statements, in order to meet Criterion 2, the therapist has to use   ACCEPTANCE   PARADOX,   SELF-DEFENSE,   and COUNTER-ATTACK.*

Patient Statement #11 I have no response to this thought that "I will be all alone if something happens to my brother."

Patient Statement #12 Isn't it true that "nobody likes me?" I can't figure out how to see it any other way.

Trainees should attempt to improvise their own responses before reading the example responses (Table 15.2)

Table 15.2 Example therapist responses: defeating negative thoughts

	Patient statement	Example therapist response
Patient statement #1	I can't seem to figure out how to challenge this thought, "Nothing will ever change."	Yeah, I can see you're feeling stuck. Can I show you how I may respond to the thought, "Nothing will ever change?" (Criterion 1) I would say something like, "Absolutely, very little really changes, what a relief, I don't have to try so hard, get my hopes up and get disappointed all the time, I can now slow down and relax!" (Criterion 2a) (Pause) OK, now can you try responding to it? (Criterion 3)
Patient statement #2	This idea has me stuck: "I have failed at everything in life."	This is a tough one, isn't it? How about I model another style, and you can see if it works for you? (Criterion 1) "The greatest success in life comes from trying and failing. I have learned tremendously from so many of my failures and will continue to learn throughout my life. My failures will be my greatest asset. So it is not a problem to have failures, merely an opportunity for growth that I can embrace." (Criterion 2a) (Pause) Now you revise that in your own words. (Criterion 3)
Patient statement #3	I just can't see how to defeat this thought, "No one understands me."	Yes, I see it's hard. How about I try to defeat it? Perhaps it will give you some ideas on how to approach it. (Criterion 1) "Absolutely, no one really understands me, I don't even understand myself sometimes, and that's OK, there's a lot that we don't understand, ultimately it's true; No one can truly understand someone standing in their separate pair of shoes." (Criterion 2a) (Pause) I see you're nodding. Did it give you a useful idea? Can you try and respond to this thought in your own words now? (Criterion 3)
Patient statement #4	I am stuck on this one: "I won't be able to cope without my husband."	It seems so real that it is difficult to challenge. Perhaps I can try and show you an alternate way to approach it. (Criterion 1) "It is true that it will be nearly impossible to cope without my husband. He did so much. It shows what a great team we were and how much I valued his support. In a way, the new challenges I have to face will be honoring his memory and the love we had. Not coping will be a wonderful opportunity that I can cherish." (Criterion 2a) (Pause) Let's see if you can put that into your own words. (Criterion 3)
Patient statement #5	I am not sure how to respond to this idea: "It's all my fault that my dad left."	I can see you're feeling stuck with it. How about I give it a try? (Criterion 1) "It may be true that my dad leaving the family had to do with me and some of my horrible behavior (Criterion 2a), at the same time he is an adult man and I was a child, he was the father and I was his kid and while sure, I wish I had been nicer, he's the father and the adult and the one responsible for his own action not just me." (Criterion 2b) (Pause) Does this give you something to work with? How about you try now responding to the negative thought in your own words? (Criterion 3)

(continued)

Table 15.2 (continued)

	Patient statement	Example therapist response
Patient statement #6	This one is just true; I can't answer that "I am going to freeze and make a fool of myself in this interview."	For sure, this is a tough one. Can I model a couple alternate ways to defeat it? (Criterion 1) "I could definitely freeze and make a fool of myself in this interview. (Criterion 2a) But that may be the best thing that can happen. First I will get an opportunity to show them that I am a genuine and open person that is okay having weaknesses and willing to take risks. Second is that I can face this fear once and for all and embrace it. In the future the idea of freezing will be no big deal. The times I freeze I will know just how to respond." (Criterion 2b) (Pause) How about you now give it a try? (Criterion 3)
Patient statement #7	I am stuck on how to respond to the thought, "Everyone is judging me because I made a mistake at work."	Yes, that's a hard one. How about I try responding to it? (Criterion 1) "Yes! People are super judgemental and quick to judge, and they are probably judging me for it. That's OK, I make mistakes all the time, and need their feedback to grow and learn. (Criterion 2a) I'm glad we have a system of checks and balances that's exactly the kind of place I want to work in. (Criterion 2a) They also probably see that I'm trying hard, that I'm eager to learn and that I care." (Criterion 2b) (Pause) Does this help? Can you try now in your own words to respond to the thought "Everyone is judging me because I made a mistake at work?"(Criterion 3)
Patient statement #8	This is hard; I don't know how to answer that "I need to be close to someone to truly be happy."	Hmm, let's brainstorm some options here. I have a couple ideas. Let me know if this resonates with you. (Criterion 1). "I can fully accept that as human beings we have a built in desire for community and connection and I am no different than anyone else. That is a beautiful thing that will continue to motivate me to work on my communication and social skills. (Criterion 2a) However this idea that I 'need' someone else to be happy just puts a lot of pressure and unrealistic expectations on both me and others. That is a lie and I am not buying into it. I can be happy on my own and this will enhance my relationship with others." (Criterion 2b). Take the parts you like and respond to that negative thought in your own words. (Criterion 3)
Patient statement #9	This one is so hard for me to challenge: "I will never get out of this rut."	I see that you're stuck. Can I try and model for you how I would respond to the thought? (Criterion 1) OK here we go: "You know what? that may be the case that I'll never completely recover from this, and will always feel depressed about it, (Criterion 2a) at the same time I'm determined to keep trying and refuse to be defeated, I have overcome difficult things before in my life, (Criterion 2b) and it's all about the way, the effort and not just about the goal. If I'm destined to live the rest of my life depressed, I can accept that too, in a way there's relief in it, life is both a gift and is hard at the same time. (Criterion 2a) I'm also kind of sick of this voice that keeps telling me things like 'I will never get out of this', I'm just going to ignore it and go about my day!" (Criterion 2c). (Pause) Do any of my arguments speak to you? Can you now give it a try? (Criterion 3)

(continued)

Table 15.2 (continued)

	Patient statement	Example therapist response
Patient statement #10	Here is the one that I get tripped up by: "I am a complete loser."	For sure, there is a block there that makes that one hard. Let me try some alternate ways to approach and you can tell me if any of them resonate with you. (Criterion 1). "There is nothing wrong with being a complete loser. I have many weaknesses and flaws and things to work on and even the best athletes lose sometimes and eventually have to retire. That is not a problem, just an opportunity. (Criterion 2a). The fact is, telling myself I am a complete loser is a ridiculous label that ignores the progress I am making and the things I do well. (Criterion 2b) The real problem is that I keep buying into the negative voice and letting it get me down. I am not doing that anymore." (Criterion 2c). (Pause) You take the parts that worked for you and put them into your own words. (Criterion 3)
Patient statement #11	I have no response to this thought that "I will be all alone if something happens to my brother."	Yes, I can see you're feeling stuck with this one. How about I give it a try? (Criterion 1) "Yes, that's totally true, I'd be devastated if I lost my brother and will feel all alone, and to a certain degree, I'll never get over that, (Criterion 2a) Nor would I actually want to get over his loss as he is so important to me. The pain will be terrible, at the same time, death is part of life, and I'll carry him with me forever (Criterion 2b) In the meantime, I just want to enjoy the time I have with him, and not listen to that fearful voice that keeps me away from being in the present moment." (Criterion 2c) Can you now give it a try? (Criterion 3)
Patient statement #12	Isn't it true that "Nobody likes me?" I can't figure out how to see it any other way.	That is a painful one, and it seems you are stuck trying to see it any other way. Let me brainstorm a few ideas for you, and you can see if any of them make sense to you. (Criterion #1). "It is completely true that I value genuine relationships. The reality is I don't like myself sometimes so it stands to reason that I won't always be likable to others. I can keep this in mind when I get together with people so I will stay motivated to be genuine and caring. (Criterion 2a) When I have done this in the past my friends and family want to spend more time with me so it is a total lie that nobody likes me. (Criterion 2b) The bigger issue is that I am listening to that negative voice. I am just not going to pay attention to it anymore and even when it does show up I will remember that those thoughts can be helpful and remind me of what is important to me." (Criterion 2c) (Pause) Take the parts that worked for you and put them into your words. (Criterion 3)

Chapter 16
Processing Learning

Skill Description

The purpose of this skill is for the patient to learn from their experience in therapy. This will increase their awareness that change is possible and achievable and that they have the tools to help themselves feel better. When a negative view of themselves or a negative thought that had been plaguing them for years is defeated, it can lead to great relief. In TEAM-CBT, this typically happens in the context of talking back to a negative thought or to a self-defeating belief using a cognitive role-play technique (see Chaps. 13 & 14). It can also happen as a result of exposure exercises, as well as addressing outcome resistance (see Chaps. 9 & 10). These moments in therapy are sometimes called "moments of enlightenment." However, as Dr. Burns often says, "we all drift in and out of enlightenment." It is almost certain that soon the relief that patients have achieved will drift away from them.

Without this technique, these moments of relief experienced in therapy may remain fleeting, left behind without a clear path to experience and access them again. Therefore, when these precious moments occur in therapy, it is important to hold on to them, emphasize them, and help etch them in our patient's memory. At that moment, the patient should slow down, take inventory, notice, and register how they are doing.[1] When patients notice that they are feeling better, it enhances their sense of positive progression and hopefulness. This can also lead to understanding what it is that got them the relief they are feeling and helping them recall it in a future moment of need. Finally, it can also help the therapist and patient decide if they are ready to tackle something else.

Therefore, when we notice relief in our patients, we want to ask questions such as:

---

[1] This is also part of the goal of using the Testing principle (Chap. 3).

M. Katz et al., *Deliberate Practice of TEAM-CBT*, SpringerBriefs in Psychology, https://doi.org/10.1007/978-3-031-46019-7_16

- What is it that you are more aware of now?
- What's changed in your thinking about this?
- What just happened right now?
- What are you thinking differently?
- What is it that was just said that clicked for you?
- What was it that made the win against the negative thought?

These questions can lead the patient to start processing what they are learning. The recommended way to use this skill is outlined in the skill criteria below. The technique concludes with asking the patient to assess how much they believe their new way of thinking to be true.

Examples of This Skill in Practice

Example #1
Patient: Wow, that totally changed things for me. It doesn't matter that I am no good. I am just a human being with flaws and failures.

Therapist: It seems like something changed for you. (Criterion 1) You said, "It doesn't matter that I am no good. I am just a human being with flaws and failures." (Criterion 2) Let's write that down. (Criterion 3) (Pause) On a scale of 0–100%, how much is this positive thought true for you right now? (Criterion 4)

Example #2
Patient: Yeah, it's true that I haven't lived up to my full potential, absolutely, and I had hoped to be more accomplished by now, and that's OK. I will continue to strive and work to improve myself, maybe for the rest of my life.

Therapist: I'm sensing you're feeling some relief? What happened there? (Criterion 1) Is it that you're accepting that there's more to accomplish and that you're happy with a life of striving and working to improve yourself? (Criterion 2) Can you write it down as a positive thought? (Criterion 3) How true is that for you, on a scale of 0–100%? (Criterion 4)

Example #3
Patient: It's not true that nobody likes me at work, and even if it was, that wouldn't be a problem because I don't need everyone to like me all the time. I am not going to buy into those negative thoughts anymore.

Therapist: Something shifted for you there. (Criterion 1) Let's see if we can capture that and write it down. (Criterion 3) You said: It's not true that nobody likes me at work, and even if it was, that wouldn't be a problem because I don't need everyone to like me all the time. I am not going to buy into those negative thoughts anymore. (Criterion 2). How much do you believe that on a scale of 0–100% right now? (Criterion 4)

Now it is your turn: Follow the Exercise Instructions and Skill Criteria (Table 16.1).

Table 16.1 Criteria for processing learning practice exercise

The therapist improvises a response to each patient statement using the following criteria:
1. Acknowledge the relief the patient is feeling.
2. Repeat or summarize the positive thought the patient said.
3. Ask the patient to write it down.
4. Ask them on a scale of 0–100% how much they believe that new positive thought to be true right now.
Proceed to the next patient statement <u>only</u> when it is too easy for the therapist to meet all criteria.

After 15 minutes of practice, the patient and therapist switch roles and start over.

Context: All patient statements occur several minutes into the second session.

Patient Statement #1 I think I see it now. It is a relief that very little really changes; I don't have to try so hard, get my hopes up, and get disappointed all the time; I can slow down and relax!

Patient Statement #2 It seems to me that the greatest success in life comes from trying and failing. So it is not a problem to have failures; it is merely an opportunity for growth that I can embrace.

Patient Statement #3 It is not a problem that no one really understands me; I don't even understand myself sometimes, and that's OK. There's a lot that we don't understand.

Patient Statement #4 It is true that it will be nearly impossible to cope without my husband. He did so much. It shows what a great team we were and how much I valued his support. In a way, the new challenges I have to face will be honoring his memory and the love we had.

Patient Statement #5 It may be true that my horrible behavior contributed to my dad leaving the family, but at the same time, he is an adult man and I was a child; he was the father and I was his kid. While I wish I had been nicer, he's the father and the adult, and the one responsible for his own actions, not just me.

Patient Statement #6 I could definitely freeze and make a fool of myself in this interview. But that may be the best thing that can happen. First, I will get an opportunity to show them that I am a genuine and open person who is okay with having weaknesses and willing to take risks. Second is that I can face this fear once and for all and embrace it. In the future, the idea of freezing will be no big deal. The times I freeze, I will know just how to respond.

Patient Statement #7   People are super judgmental and quick to judge, and they are probably judging me for it. That's OK, I make mistakes all the time and need their feedback to grow and learn. I'm glad we have a system of checks and balances, that's exactly the kind of place I want to work in. They also probably see that I'm trying hard, that I'm eager to learn and that I care.

Patient Statement #8   I can fully accept that as human beings we have a built-in desire for community and connection and I am no different than anyone else. That is a beautiful thing that will continue to motivate me to work on my communication and social skills. However, this idea that I "need" someone else to be happy just puts a lot of pressure and unrealistic expectations on both me and others. That is a lie, and I am not buying into it. I can be happy on my own and this will enhance my relationship with others.

Patient Statement #9   You know what? That may be the case that I'll never completely recover from this and will always feel depressed about it, but at the same time, I'm determined to keep trying and refuse to be defeated. I have overcome difficult things before in my life, and it's all about the way, the effort, and not just about the goal. If I'm destined to live the rest of my life depressed, I can accept that too. In a way, there's relief in it; life is both a gift and hard at the same time. I'm also kind of sick of this voice that keeps telling me things like "I will never get out of this", I'm just going to ignore it and go about my day!

Patient Statement #10   There is nothing wrong with being a complete loser. I have many weaknesses and flaws and things to work on, and even the best athletes lose sometimes and eventually have to retire. That is not a problem, just an opportunity. The fact is, telling myself I am a complete loser is a ridiculous label that ignores the progress I am making and the things I do well. The real problem is that I keep buying into the negative voice and letting it get me down. I am not doing that anymore.

Patient Statement #11   Yes, that's totally true. I'd be devastated if I lost my brother and would feel all alone, and to a certain degree, I'll never get over that, nor would I actually want to get over his loss as he is so important to me. The pain will be terrible, but at the same time, death is part of life, and I'll carry him with me forever. In the meantime, I just want to enjoy the time I have with him and not listen to that fearful voice that keeps me away from being in the present moment.

Patient Statement #12   It is completely true that I value genuine relationships. The reality is that I don't like myself sometimes, so it stands to reason that I won't always be likeable to others. I can keep this in mind when I get together with people, so I will stay motivated to be genuine and caring. When I have done this in the past, my friends and family want to spend more time with me, so it is a total lie that nobody likes me. The bigger issue is that I am listening to that negative voice. I am just not going to pay attention to it anymore, and even when it does show up, I will remember that those thoughts can be helpful and remind me of what is important to me.

Trainees should attempt to improvise their own responses before reading the example responses (Table 16.2)

Table 16.2 Example therapist responses: processing learning

	Patient statement	Example therapist response
Patient statement #1	I think I see it now. It is a relief that very little really changes; I don't have to try so hard, get my hopes up, and get disappointed all the time; I can slow down and relax!	Ah, I can sense a little relief in you. (Criterion 1) You don't have to try so hard, you can just slow down and relax. (Criterion 2) Can you write it down? (Criterion 3) On a scale of 0–100%, how much do you believe that you don't need to try so hard, and that you can relax and slow down? (Criterion 4)
Patient statement #2	It seems to me that the greatest success in life comes from trying and failing. So it is not a problem to have failures; it is merely an opportunity for growth that I can embrace.	That is quite a change in perspective. (Criterion 1) So, you are saying that failing is a good thing because it provides opportunities for growth and learning. (Criterion 2). Let's write that down. (Criterion 3) On a scale of 0–100%, how true is that for you? (Criterion 4)
Patient statement #3	It is not a problem that no one really understands me; I don't even understand myself sometimes, and that's OK. There's a lot that we don't understand.	Yeah, I can see you're feeling some relief, is that right? (Criterion 1) No one really understands, and no one needs to understand me for it to be OK. (Criterion 2) Can you write it down? (Criterion 3) On a scale of 0–100%, how much do you believe that even if no one really understands you, it's OK? (Criterion 4)
Patient statement #4	It is true that it will be nearly impossible to cope without my husband. He did so much. It shows what a great team we were and how much I valued his support. In a way, the new challenges I have to face will be honoring his memory and the love we had.	There seems to be a shift in your thinking. (Criterion 1) I heard you say that not being able to cope will be honoring his memory, demonstrating the love you had for each other and what a great team you were. (Criterion 2) Let's write that down. (Criterion 3) On a scale of 0–100%, how much is that true for you? (Criterion 4)
Patient statement #5	It may be true that my horrible behavior contributed to my dad leaving the family, but at the same time he is an adult man and I was a child; he was the father and I was his kid. While I wish I had been nicer, he's the father and the adult, and the one responsible for his own actions, not just me.	Exactly! I love that! You seem to be realizing something important here, is that right? (Criterion 1) Ultimately, you were just a child, and your dad was the adult, and he, not you, was responsible for his decisions. (Criterion 2) Can you write it down? (Criterion 3) Now, on a scale of 0–100%, how much do you believe that it is your father and not you, that's responsible for his decision to leave? (Criterion 4)

(continued)

Table 16.2 (continued)

	Patient statement	Example therapist response
Patient statement #6	I could definitely freeze and make a fool of myself in this interview. But that may be the best thing that can happen. First, I will get an opportunity to show them that I am a genuine and open person who is okay with having weaknesses and willing to take risks. Second is that I can face this fear once and for all and embrace it. In the future, the idea of freezing will be no big deal. The times I freeze, I will know just how to respond.	Something changed for you there. (Criterion 1) I heard you say that freezing in an interview is no big deal; it will give you an opportunity to face that fear head-on and know how to respond in the future. In addition, freezing will reveal your genuineness, openness, and that you are okay with having weaknesses and taking risks. (Criterion 2) Let's write that down. (Criterion 3) How much do you believe that, on a 0–100 scale? (Criterion 4)
Patient statement #7	People are super judgmental and quick to judge, and they are probably judging me for it. That's OK, I make mistakes all the time and need their feedback to grow and learn. I'm glad we have a system of checks and balances, that's exactly the kind of place I want to work in. They also probably see that I'm trying hard, that I'm eager to learn and that I care.	I'm sensing that you're feeling better about this, is that right? (Criterion 1) That it's OK to be judged, and make mistakes cause it's the only way to grow and learn; it's almost like it's a privilege to be in a system that evaluates you and points out where you need to improve. (Criterion 2) Is that right? Can you write it down? (Criterion 3) On a scale of 0–100%, how much do you believe that it's OK to be in a system where you're judged and getting feedback just so you can learn and grow? (Criterion 4)
Patient statement #8	I can fully accept that, as human beings we have a built-in desire for community and connection, and I am no different than anyone else. That is a beautiful thing that will continue to motivate me to work on my communication and social skills. However, this idea that I "need" someone else to be happy just puts a lot of pressure and unrealistic expectations on both me and others. That is a lie, and I am not buying into it. I can be happy on my own, and this will enhance my relationship with others.	I am noticing a relief in your voice. What changed for you there? (Criterion 1) You said a couple of things. First, you can fully accept yourself as a human being with a desire for connection and community, which is a beautiful thing. Second, you are no longer buying into the idea that you "need" others, because that puts too much pressure and unrealistic expectations on you. In fact, you can be happy on your own, which will enhance your other relationships. (Criterion 2) Let's write this down. (Criterion 3) On a 0–100% scale, how true is this? (Criterion 4)

(continued)

Table 16.2 (continued)

	Patient statement	Example therapist response
Patient statement #9	You know what? That may be the case that I'll never completely recover from this, and will always feel depressed about it, but at the same time, I'm determined to keep trying and refuse to be defeated. I have overcome difficult things before in my life, and it's all about the way, the effort, and not just about the goal. If I'm destined to live the rest of my life depressed, I can accept that too. In a way, there's relief in it; life is both a gift and hard at the same time. I'm also kind of sick of this voice that keeps telling me things like "I will never get out of this", I'm just going to ignore it and go about my day!	Love it! It's like you're experiencing a little bit of enlightenment right now, right? (Criterion 1) I love what you're saying, can you write it down? (Criterion 3) "Ignore it and go about my day!" (Criterion 2) How much, on a scale of 0-100, do you believe that it's all about the way and that life is both a gift and hard at the same time? (Criterion 4)
Patient statement #10	There is nothing wrong with being a complete loser. I have many weaknesses and flaws and things to work on, and even the best athletes lose sometimes and eventually have to retire. That is not a problem, just an opportunity. The fact is, telling myself I am a complete loser is a ridiculous label that ignores the progress I am making and the things I do well. The real problem is that I keep buying into the negative voice and letting it get me down. I am not doing that anymore.	I am sensing a significant feeling of relief in you with your response. (Criterion 1) I heard you say three things. One, losing or being a loser is just an acknowledgment that you have weaknesses and flaws, which present an opportunity for growth. Second, that you do well in many things and are making progress, so the label of a complete loser is ridiculous. Third, the real problem is buying into the negative voice, and you are not going to do that anymore. (Criterion 2) Take a moment to write that down. (Criterion 3) How much do you believe on a scale of 0-100? (Criterion 4)
Patient statement #11	Yes, that's totally true. I'd be devastated if I lost my brother and would feel all alone, and to a certain degree, I'll never get over that, nor would I actually want to get over his loss as he is so important to me. The pain will be terrible, but at the same time, death is part of life, and I'll carry him with me forever. In the meantime, I just want to enjoy the time I have with him and not listen to that fearful voice that keeps me away from being in the present moment.	Ugh, it's so sad, and I also sense the relief in what you're saying. (Criterion 1) that the pain of losing your brother will be terrible, but in a way, that's how you'd want it to be. (Criterion 2) Can you write this down? (Criterion 3) On a scale of 0–100, how much do you believe it to be true that it will be terrible and that you'll carry him with you, and ultimately you wouldn't want it any other way? (Criterion 4)

(continued)

Table 16.2 (continued)

	Patient statement	Example therapist response
Patient statement #12	It is completely true that I value genuine relationships. The reality is that I don't like myself sometimes so it stands to reason that I won't always be likeable to others. I can keep this in mind when I get together with people, so I will stay motivated to be genuine and caring. When I have done this in the past, my friends and family want to spend more time with me so it is a total lie that nobody likes me. The bigger issue is that I am listening to that negative voice. I am just not going to pay attention to it anymore, and even when it does show up I will remember that those thoughts can be helpful and remind me of what is important to me.	There is a change in your thinking that appears to be giving you tremendous relief. (Criterion 1) You said: It is completely true that you value genuine relationships. The reality is that you don't like yourself sometimes, so it stands to reason that you won't always be likeable to others. Keeping this in mind will motivate you to be genuine and caring. When you have done this in the past, your friends and family want to spend more time with you, so it is a total lie that nobody likes you. You are not going to pay attention to the negative voice anymore, and even when it does show up, you will remember that those thoughts can be helpful and remind you of what is important. (Criterion 2) Let's write that down. (Criterion 3) How true is that for you on a 0–100% scale? (Criterion 4)

Chapter 17
Assigning Homework

Skill Description

TEAM-CBT provides a roadmap (Table 17.1) for therapists with a series of sequential steps toward overcoming mental health suffering. Homework is used to practice new skills, connect in-between sessions, and help move therapy forward toward the next sequential step. Therapy homework is seen as integral and necessary toward the process of recovery. We spend a good amount of time educating the patient about expectations for homework and holding them accountable for it.

Two kinds of therapy homework are typically assigned at each session: (Table 17.1)

1. Lifestyle/wellbeing-related homework. This includes regular exercise, sleep hygiene, and meditation. This homework is typically behavioral in nature.
2. Therapy process-specific homework. Since TEAM-CBT is a series of sequential steps, we can use homework to prepare the patient and start to move toward the next step in the therapy process. This homework is typically cognitive in nature.

Good homework tasks make sense given the current stage of the therapy process, flow easily into our patient's life, and make our patient feel excited about doing them.

Each therapy session starts with a review of current mood (Exercise 1), feedback on previous sessions, and a brief review of previous homework assignments.[1] Homework is often assigned throughout the session, and each session ends with reviewing homework for the following session.

The focus on homework usually begins during the very first encounter with our patient, even prior to the intake session. In addition to reviewing and assigning homework each session, sometimes parts of the session are dedicated to creating

---

[1] Following up on homework in the next session is a challenge worth practicing and thinking about. It is beyond the scope of this book.

© The Author(s), under exclusive license to Springer Nature Switzerland AG 2023   117
M. Katz et al., *Deliberate Practice of TEAM-CBT*, SpringerBriefs in Psychology,
https://doi.org/10.1007/978-3-031-46019-7_17

Table 17.1 Homework flow

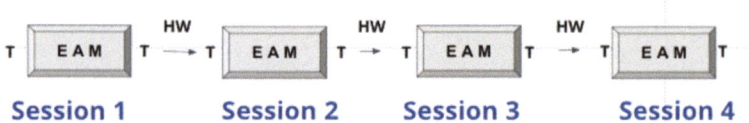

| Session 1 | Session 2 | Session 3 | Session 4 |

Table 17.2 Roadmap of TEAM-CBT process

Testing/empathy	Invitation	Specificity	Conceptualization	Outcome resistance	Process resistance	Methods

accountability and setting expectations for homework. Often techniques such as the gentle ultimatum (Exercise 7A and 7B) are used to remove barriers against doing homework, by writing out the advantages of NOT doing homework.

As the last skill in this book, this exercise serves two purposes for the reader:

1. Practice assigning relevant homework to patients that moves the therapy forward.
2. An opportunity to internalize the TEAM-CBT roadmap.

When new to TEAM-CBT, therapists tend to assign homework that is nonspecific to the step in therapy they are in (Empathy, Invitation, Specificity, Conceptualization, Outcome Resistance, Process Resistance, Methods) (Table 17.2). Rather, you will likely gravitate prematurely to assigning homework from the Methods step. In this exercise, we ask you to take note of which step in TEAM-CBT you are in for each patient scenario and choose a homework assignment that is relevant to that step as outlined in Table 17.3.

Examples of This Skill in Practice

Note: The patient should read aloud the context information provided and where they are on the TEAM-CBT road map. All patient contexts occur during the last 10 minutes of a session.

Example #1

Context: You have a new patient who just accepted an invitation to work on depression. The next step is *specificity*.

Testing	Invitation	**Specificity**	Conceptualization	Outcome resistance	Process resistance	Methods

Table 17.3 Suggested homework tasks based on where you are at in the TEAM-CBT process

TEAM-step	Conceptualization	Patient homework tasks examples
Testing/empathy	Undecided yet	Testing: "Brief Mood Survey," "Concept of Self Help," and "How to Make Therapy Rewarding and Successful" memos. Journaling, writing out goals for therapy.
Invitation/specificity	Depression	Capture a moment in time you when were feeling depressed.
	Anxiety	Capture a moment in time when you were feeling anxious.
	Habit/addiction	Capture a moment in time when you will be feeling tempted.
	Relationship problem	Capture interaction you did not feel good about.
Addressing outcome resistance	Depression	Create a table of advantages and disadvantages for feeling depressed or write out the good values feeling depressed shows about you and the true benefits it brings to your life.
	Anxiety	Create a table of advantages and disadvantages for feeling anxious or write out the good values feeling anxious shows about you and the true benefits it brings to your life.
	Habit/addiction	Create a three-column table with three kinds of advantages the habit brings to your life: the good values having the habit shows about you, the benefits of the habit to your life, and what you stand to lose if you stop the habit completely. Create a table with advantages and disadvantages of sobriety.
	Relationship problem	Create a table with the advantages of resolving the problems and getting closer to the other person, vs. creating healthier boundaries or distance from them, vs. staying the status quo (Interpersonal Decision Making Form.)
Addressing process Resistance	Depression	Create a table of advantages and disadvantages for doing the work necessary to overcome depression.
	Anxiety	Create a table of advantages and disadvantages for doing exposure therapy.
	Habit/addiction	Create a table of advantages and disadvantages for doing homework, getting started on tasks, going to 12-step meetings, or committing to accountability steps.
	Relationship problem	Create a table of the advantages and disadvantages of blaming the other person for problems in your relationship.

(continued)

Table 17.3 (continued)

TEAM-step	Conceptualization	Patient homework tasks examples
Methods	Depression	Examine the evidence. Identify the distortions.
	Anxiety	Exposure exercises.
	Habit/addiction	Self-disclosure with friends and family members. Write down and challenge tempting thoughts with self-control thoughts.
	Relationship problem	Write out revised responses to moments in which you did not communicate well. Practice five secrets of effective communication with friends and colleagues.

Therapist: [Mental note: Specificity (Criterion 1)] Let's talk about homework that could help you. (Criterion 2) I suggest you take a few moments every day to write down a specific moment in time when you were feeling depressed. When was it, who was with you, and two columns: one for your thoughts and one for your feelings in that moment. (Criterion 3) Would you be willing to do that? If so, for how many times per week? (Criterion 4)

Example #2

Context: You have been working with a software engineer who is feeling depressed after recently losing their job. During this session, you've started a table to address *outcome resistance* (Exercise 6B). This table is a cost–benefit analysis where the patient has just started to list the advantages of being depressed for losing their job. As the session time is running out, the next step is to set up homework for the patient to continue this work.

Testing	Invitation	Specificity	Conceptualization	**Outcome resistance**	Process resistance	Methods

Therapist: [Mental note: Outcome resistance (Criterion 1)] I'm noticing the time; let's decide on what you can do between now and our next session. (Criterion 2) How about, as the first part of your homework, adding at least 3–5 more benefits and values for depression to the table we started. (Criterion 3) Would you be willing to commit to spending at least 10 minutes doing this before the end of the day today? (Criterion 4)

Example #3

Context: It's 7 minutes before the end of the third session with a patient. You and your patient are working on improving their relationships with colleagues. During the session, you reviewed the Five Secrets for Effective Communication (Exercise 2A and 2B). A good next step may be to set up the patient to practice the Five Secrets for Effective Communication at home.

Testing	Invitation	Specificity	Conceptualization	Outcome resistance	Process resistance	**Methods**

Therapist: [Mental note: Methods (Criteria 1)] Let's talk about where to take it from here, and what you can do between now and our next session. (Criterion 2) How about practicing each of the five secrets, two days at a time? For example, make today and tomorrow "Thought Empathy" days, and start every interaction with people in your life first by repeating some of what they said verbatim? (Criterion 3) Are you willing to commit to working on this for 15 minutes a day every day this week? (Criterion 4)

> **Now it is your turn: Follow the Exercise Instructions and Skill Criteria (Table 17.4).**

> **After 15 minutes of practice, the patient and therapist switch roles and start over.**

Note: The patient should read aloud the context information provided and where they are on the TEAM CBT roadmap. All patient contexts occur during the last 10 minutes of a session.

Patient Context #1

The patient wants to work on depression. You have focused on a specific event during which they have felt depressed, and have addressed outcome and process resistance. They have chosen that thought: "I should be better than this by now." The session has a few minutes left. More cognitive techniques are needed to overcome this negative thought.

Testing	Invitation	Specificity	Conceptualization	Outcome resistance	Process resistance	**Methods**

Table 17.4 Criteria for processing learning practice exercise

The therapist improvises a response to each patient statement using the following criteria:
1. Make a mental note of the TEAM-CBT step you are in and state it out loud.
2. Redirect the conversation to wrapping up and homework.
3. Assign homework that is relevant to the TEAM CBT step and is applicable to the problem the patient is facing.
4. Ask the patient for details regarding their commitment to completing the homework (e.g., when they will do it, how they will do it, how often, where, and for how long?).
Proceed to the next patient statement only when it is too easy for the therapist to meet all criteria.

Patient Context #2

During a 15-minute pretherapy consultation, the patient indicates that they want help to overcome social anxiety. In preparation for your intake session, you explain the purpose of the testing forms. Now it's time to have them fill out the testing forms.

Testing	Invitation	Specificity	Conceptualization	Outcome resistance	Process resistance	Methods

Patient Context #3

The patient wants help with a strained relationship with their boss. You've identified the focus of the work is on the relationship problem, addressed outcome and process resistance, and introduced the five secrets for effective communication to them. Now it's time to improve their communication skills.

Testing	Invitation	Specificity	Conceptualization	Outcome resistance	Process resistance	**Methods**

Patient Context #4

The patient wants help with their habit of drinking alcohol every night, and you've identified removing all alcohol from the household as their first target. You've addressed outcome and process resistance and decided the patient will free their home from alcohol tonight. Now is the time to have them clear their home and report back to you that they did it.

Testing	Invitation	Specificity	Conceptualization	Outcome resistance	Process resistance	**Methods**

Patient Context #5

The patient asks for help with the relationship with their teenage son who is struggling with addiction. You have empathized and offered an invitation. The patient is unsure about their goals for the relationship. The next step is to set up homework to address outcome resistance.

Testing	Invitation	Specificity	Conceptualization	**Outcome resistance**	Process resistance	Methods

Patient Context #6

The patient identified wanting help with their alcohol habit. However, you haven't addressed outcome resistance yet. Setting up a cost–benefit analysis uncovering the benefits of continuing to drink is next (Exercise 6B).

Testing	Invitation	Specificity	Conceptualization	**Outcome resistance**	Process resistance	Methods

Patient Context #7

You are working with a patient to address their anxiety about parenting. During the session, you completed the positive reframe table together and came up with all the benefits and values of feeling anxious. The next step is reviewing those advantages, considering if there are any disadvantages, and writing those down.

Testing	Invitation	Specificity	Conceptualization	**Outcome resistance**	Process resistance	Methods

Patient Context #8

You have a depressed patient asking for help with feeling defective, down, and guilty. He states that he has a tough time getting out of bed in the morning because he feels unmotivated and is unsure about doing homework. The next step is to set up an experiment where he stays in bed one day, the next day gets up at 8 am, and at noon every day he tracks how he feels about himself.

Testing	Invitation	Specificity	Conceptualization	Outcome resistance	**Process resistance**	Methods

Patient Context #9

The patient is in therapy to get help with depression and hopelessness. You have worked through the agenda-setting steps and been trying a few cognitive methods. The patient is stuck on the thought, "I will never get over this." You identify that there is still some lingering outcome resistance with depression and hopelessness. The next step is to revisit the motivation using a CBA with the thought.

Testing	Invitation	Specificity	Conceptualization	**Outcome resistance**	Process resistance	Methods

Patient Context #10

The patient wishes to get help improving his relationship with his partner. You haven't addressed resistance with him yet. Now it's time to address the relationship's outcome resistance using a cost–benefit analysis comparing the advantages of becoming more intimate and close with his partner, staying in the status quo, or creating a safer distance from them.

Testing	Invitation	Specificity	Conceptualization	**Outcome resistance**	Process resistance	Methods

Patient Context #11

The patient is a college student who has accepted the invitation to get to work on procrastination. You have identified that the specific moment in time they struggle is sitting down in the evening to play video games instead of working on his course project. The next step is to address outcome resistance by having her complete a cost–benefit analysis table for it.

Testing	Invitation	Specificity	Conceptualization	**Outcome resistance**	Process resistance	Methods

Patient Context #12

The whole session was spent on empathy. All invitations were refused for more empathy. You haven't been able to focus using invitation and specificity (Exercises 4 and 5). The next step is for the patient to journal and record difficult or challenging moments and reflect on what they may want help with.

Testing	**Invitation**	Specificity	Conceptualization	Outcome resistance	Process resistance	Methods

Patient Context #13

You have a depressed patient asking for help with feeling inadequate, lonely, and sad. He states that he is feeling too hopeless, and unsure if he can do much homework. The next step is to create a table with the advantages and disadvantages of feeling hopeless.

Testing	Invitation	Specificity	Conceptualization	Outcome resistance	**Process resistance**	Methods

Trainees should attempt to improvise their own responses before reading the example responses (Table 17.5)

Table 17.5 Example therapist responses: assigning homework

	Patient context	Example therapist response
Patient context #1	The patient wants to work on depression. You have focused on a specific event during which they have felt depressed, and have addressed outcome and process resistance. They have chosen that thought: "I should be better than this by now." The session has a few minutes left. More cognitive techniques are needed to overcome this negative thought.	Mental note: Methods. The step we are in is Methods. (Criterion 1) Let's transition into figuring out how to move forward between now and our next session. (Criterion 2) Please put the thought "I should be better than this by now" on the top of a page and use the following techniques with it: 1. Identify the distortions based on the list you have. 2. Respond to this negative thought with your positive voice, in writing, using self-defense, acceptance paradox, and counterattack approaches. (Criterion 3) Is there anything else you'd like to add as your homework? When would you commit to tackling this? (Criterion 4)
Patient context #2	During a 15-minute pretherapy consultation the patient indicates that they want help to overcome social anxiety. In preparation for your intake session, you explain the purpose of the testing forms. Now it's time to have them fill out the testing forms.	Mental note: Testing. The step we are in is Testing. (Criterion 1) Let's clarify the next steps in preparing for our intake session. (Criterion 2) There are three forms for you to fill out that will maximize the effectiveness of our work together. Before and after every session, you will fill out a brief mood survey, and prior to our first session, there are two memos that will clarify our expectations for each other and help us to identify anything that might get in the way of your goals for therapy. (Criterion 3). It is important for those to be done before our intake session. What day are you planning to complete them? (Criterion 4)
Patient context #3	The patient wants help with a strained relationship with their boss. You've identified the focus of the work is on the relationship problem, addressed outcome and process resistance, and introduced the five secrets for effective communication to them. Now it's time to improve their communication skills.	Mental note: Methods The step we are in is Methods. (Criterion 1) Here's what I suggest you do for homework. (Criterion 2) Read *Feeling Good Together* for 40 minutes per day and practice using the exercises in the book. (Criterion 3) Is that something you can commit too? When would you do it in your day? for how many days per week? (Criterion 4)

(continued)

Table 17.5 (continued)

	Patient context	Example therapist response
Patient context #4	The patient wants help with their habit of drinking alcohol every night, and you've identified removing all alcohol from the household as their first target. You've addressed outcome and process resistance and decided the patient will free their home from alcohol tonight. Now is the time to have them clear their home and report back to you that they did it.	Mental note: Methods The step we are in is Methods. (Criterion 1) That is great to hear. You will do whatever takes. Here is your homework. (Criterion 2) When you get home from work tonight, you are going to get rid of all the alcohol in your home, then send me a text when you are done. (Criterion 3). Are you willing to do that, and what time can I expect your text? (Criterion 4)
Patient context #5	The patient asks for help with the relationship with their teenage son who is struggling with addiction. You have empathized and offered an invitation. The patient is unsure about their goals for the relationship. The next step is to set up homework to address outcome resistance.	Mental note: Outcome Resistance The step we are in is Outcome Resistance. (Criterion 1) Let's pause here and think about the next steps for you to take before our next session. (Criterion 2) Let's create a table together listing the advantages of the three options you have in this case: (1) Advantages of getting closer with your son, as difficult as it may be. (2) Advantages of keeping the status quo with your son for now, that's the path of least resistance. (3) Advantages of creating a safer and greater distance from your son. (Criterion 3) Can you do that? I'd like to devote 30-45 minutes to this task, so you could really do it thoroughly and thoughtfully. Is that OK with you? (Criterion 4)
Patient context #6	The patient identified wanting help with their alcohol habit. However, you haven't addressed outcome resistance yet. Setting up a cost–benefit analysis uncovering the benefits of continuing to drink is next (Exercise 6B).	Mental note: Outcome Resistance The step we are in is Outcome Resistance. (Criterion 1) Let's think about your homework for this week. (Criterion 2). I want you to complete this cost–benefit analysis and explore the benefits of continuing to drink. (Criterion 3) Can you commit to speeding 10 minutes a day for 5 days this week filling out the CBA and identifying all the advantages and disadvantages of drinking? (Criterion 4)

(continued)

Table 17.5 (continued)

	Patient context	Example therapist response
Patient context #7	You are working with a patient to address their anxiety about parenting. During the session you completed the positive reframe table together and came up with all the benefits and values of feeling anxious. The next step is reviewing those advantages, considering if there are any disadvantages, and writing those down.	Mental note: Outcome Resistance The step we are in is Outcome Resistance. (Criterion 1) So let's change gears, and set up the work to do between now and our next session. (Criterion 2) I'd like you to take each of those advantages of feeling anxious, and write a response to each one of them. To do that, make them into a devil's advocate statement like "Anxiety shows you care, so it's important you keep on being anxious!", then respond to this devil's advocate statement in writing. You should end up with a few pages of paragraphs, each starting with a devil's advocate statement and followed by a robust response to it. (Criterion 3) This will take 60–90 minutes to complete. Is that something you could commit to doing? (Criterion 4)
Patient context #8	You have a depressed patient asking for help with feeling defective, down, and guilty. He states that he has a tough time getting out of bed in the morning because he feels unmotivated and is unsure about doing homework. The next step is to set up an experiment where he stays in bed one day, the next day gets up at 8 am, and at noon every day he tracks how he feels about himself.	Mental note: Process Resistance (Criterion 1) The step we are in is Process Resistance. (Criterion 1) Before we begin wrapping up today, let's talk about the homework plan. (Criterion 2) This week let's try an experiment to see if it makes sense for you to get up and do the homework even when you don't feel like it. I want you to alternate with one day you stay in bed and the next day you get up at 8 am. At noon every day, make a note about how you are feeling on a 0–10 scale. (Criterion 3) Are you able to commit to that experiment and follow through every day? (Criterion 4)
Patient context #9	The patient is in therapy to get help with depression and hopelessness. You have worked through the agenda setting steps and been trying a few cognitive methods. The patient is stuck on the thought, "I will never get over this." You identify that there is still some lingering outcome resistance with depression and hopelessness. The next step is to revisit the motivation using a CBA with the thought.	Mental note: Outcome Resistance The step we are in is Outcome Resistance. (Criterion 1) Let's pause here and think about therapy homework. (Criterion 2) Can you write the thought "believing I will never get over this" on the top of a page, divide it into two columns, one side for advantages, the other disadvantages? Now, as homework, can you fill out the table with the advantages and disadvantages of believing that thought? (Criterion 3) Can you devote 20 minutes to doing it? (Criterion 4)

(continued)

Table 17.5 (continued)

	Patient context	Example therapist response
Patient context #10	The patient wishes to get help improving his relationship with his partner. You haven't addressed resistance with him yet. Now it's time to address the relationship's outcome resistance using a cost–benefit analysis, comparing the advantages of becoming more intimate and close with his partner, staying the status quo or creating a safer distance from them.	Mental note: Outcome Resistance (Criterion 1) The step we are in is Outcome Resistance. (Criterion 1) Okay, why don't we take a minute to clarify the homework plan for this week. (Criterion 1) Before we jump into communication skills, it is important to explore what it is you are really wanting in this relationship. Take three sheets of paper and do a cost–benefit analysis for these three options: 1. Getting closer and building intimacy with your partner 2. Keeping your relationship the same as it is right now 3. Creating a safer distance from your partner. (Criterion 3) Can you commit to working on this for 15 minutes a day every day this week? (Criterion 4)
Patient context #11	The patient wishes to get help improving his relationship with his partner. You haven't addressed resistance with him yet. Now it's time to address the relationship's outcome resistance using a cost–benefit analysis comparing the advantages of becoming more intimate and close with his partner, staying in the status quo, or creating a safer distance from them.	Mental note: Outcome Resistance for procrastination The step we are in is Outcome Resistance. (Criterion 1) Let's think about how to move this forward between sessions. (Criterion 2) Can you write "Procrastination/Postponing things" At the top of a page, divide it into two columns: one for advantages, one for disadvantages? Now for homework, please write out the beautiful values and advantages that postponing things shows about you, without any cynicism, as well as the disadvantages of postponing things. (Criterion 3) Can you spend 20 minutes on this perhaps right now after our session? (Criterion 4)
Patient context #12	The whole session was spent on empathy. All invitations were refused for more empathy. You haven't been able to focus using invitation and specificity (Exercises 4 and 5). The next step is for the patient to journal and record difficult or challenging moments and reflect on what they may want help with.	Mental note: Invitation. The step we are in is Invitation. (Criterion 1) Let's pause for a moment and think about the homework you can do to clarify our goals for therapy. (Criterion 2) Every evening, think about your day and write down in your journal a difficult or challenging moment. Before our next session, consider whether or not you would like some help with it. (Criterion 3) Can you commit to doing that every evening this week? (Criterion 4)

(continued)

Table 17.5 (continued)

	Patient context	Example therapist response
Patient context #13	You have a depressed patient asking for help with feeling inadequate, lonely, and sad. He states that he is feeling too hopeless, and unsure if he can do much homework. The next step is to create a table with the advantages and disadvantages of feeling hopeless.	Mental note: Process Resistance. The step we are in is Process Resistance. (Criterion 1) I can sense your hopelessness and that's very important as we think about next steps. Feeling hopeless is an important feeling to focus on. (Criterion 2) To get it started, please take out a piece of paper and divide it into two, on one side write "advantages" and on the other "disadvantages." Now, on the top write "Feeling Hopeless." Would you be willing to devote 15–20 minutes to this cost–benefit analysis for feeling hopeless before our next session? (Criterion 3 and 4)

Part III
Example Session Transcript
and Conclusion

Chapter 18
Annotated Session Transcript

So far, you have been learning and practicing isolated clinical skills. We will now pull these together by showing how these skills can be used in a real-world clinical session. The annotated transcript below demonstrates how clinical skills can be flexibly integrated in a manner that is both technically rigorous and responsive to the patient's statements and needs.

We recommend reading through the transcript carefully. Reflect on how and why skills were used in certain contexts. We also recommend that you take this opportunity to reflect on which specific skills demonstrated here warrant further deliberate practice on your part. Remember, reading and studying transcripts can be very helpful for your professional development, especially if it informs further skill rehearsal!

Annotated Transcript

This session was conducted at a TEAM-CBT conference with a workshop member who volunteered for personal work in a live therapy demonstration. I (Mike) and my colleague Heather were co-therapists working with Kevin. Kevin had already done a fair amount of homework for us. Before our meeting, he filled out a brief mood survey and daily mood log.

Heather (therapist): So, how are you doing right now, Kevin? (Inquiry: Chap. 5)

Kevin (patient): I'm a little nervous. The workshop this morning definitely was a good warm-up, so I'm less nervous than I would have naturally been.

Heather (therapist): Well, thanks for sharing that. I'm pretty nervous too, actually. ("I Feel" Statements: Chap. 5)

Mike (therapist): Would it be OK if we were all nervous together for a little bit? ("I Feel" Statements and Inquiry: Chap. 5)

Kevin (patient): I think so, yeah.

© The Author(s), under exclusive license to Springer Nature Switzerland AG 2023
M. Katz et al., *Deliberate Practice of TEAM-CBT*, SpringerBriefs in Psychology,
https://doi.org/10.1007/978-3-031-46019-7_18

Heather (therapist): So Kevin, looking at your "Brief Mood Survey" (BMS) here, I can see that you're reporting feeling somewhat sad and discouraged and a loss of motivation for things. No loss of pleasure in your life, but a moderate feeling of low self-esteem or worthlessness. And I see that you're not having any suicidal thoughts or urges. (Chap. 3: Testing) For the anxiety you scored, feeling a lot anxious, a lot tense, and on edge. Moderately frightened and worried about things and extremely nervous. So that's a pretty high score for the anxiety cluster. And for the anger/frustration section, the only thing you checked was feeling somewhat frustrated. The happiness score is pretty high. You feel a lot happy and joyful, motivated, and productive. You feel extremely hopeful and optimistic and extreme for pleasure and satisfaction in life. But only moderate for feeling worthwhile and high self-esteem. And you marked that you did a lot of homework. Thank you so much for sharing all that with us. (Chap. 3: Testing)

Kevin (patient): Of course.

Heather (therapist): I'd like to invite you to fill us in and tell us a little bit about what's going on and what you'd like help with. (Inquiry: Chap. 5)

Kevin (patient): I guess I have a very low social battery. So I force myself to be really social, but I'm really more of an introverted person. And then I start burning out and I can see that. I feel to some extent that I overcompensate and then it's a hard crash. Then I get worried that when that sociable person kind of goes away, people might think that I wasn't being authentic or that I'm bipolar, even.

Heather (therapist): So, what I'm hearing is that you describe yourself as having a low social battery. And I think you said that you will push yourself, you'll overcompensate and then get to a state of feeling kind of burned out. And then you worry that people will judge you if they see that, and see you as inauthentic or maybe even bipolar. (Though Empathy: Chap. 4) And I can imagine this would make you feel anxious and worried. Maybe also frustrated. Maybe also feel kind of sad or insecure. (Feeling Empathy: Chap. 4)

Kevin (patient): Yeah.

Heather (therapist): Maybe other feelings that I haven't mentioned? Can you tell us more what it's been like for you? (Inquiry: Chap. 5)

Kevin (patient): Yeah, there's a sense of overwhelm with the overcompensating and trying to be extra social and then, afterwards, trying to maintain that. And even just process what people I talk to, who I met, you know, if I'm just meeting a bunch of people.

Mike (therapist): Kevin, I'm just appreciating your openness with us right now here in front of everyone. (Stroking: Chap. 5) And I heard you say that there's a sense of, with that extra social interaction, a kind of an overwhelm. (Thought Empathy: Chap. 4) And when you have to maintain that, I imagine it must be exhausting at times. (Feeling Empathy: Chap. 4) Is it? (Inquiry: Chap. 5)

Kevin (patient): Yeah. Like this week, it's been great and there's that conflict of like, I love meeting new people and socializing, but then three days in I'm completely burnt out and running on fumes.

Mike (therapist): So, there is this excitement about being here and really wanting to be here, but after three days of really putting yourself out there, the sense of burnout and overwhelm and exhaustion all at the same time. Yeah, and you're feeling some of that even right now. (Feeling Empathy: Chap. 4)

Kevin (patient): And there's also a bit of shame, cause most people don't see that part of me. You know, I just did some shame-attacking exercises and I was doing crazy stuff. I feel like nobody would believe me if I said that I'm kind of burning out, you know?

Heather (therapist): I felt moved to hear you say that. (I Feel Statements: Chap. 5) But most people don't see this part of you. So, after seeing you engaging in shame attacking, they might not believe that this is such a struggle for you. (Thought Empathy: Chap. 4) I can imagine feeling very alone, or not being seen, or misunderstood. (Feeling Empathy: Chap. 4)

Kevin (patient): Yeah, yeah, there is a loneliness with that. Almost like a disconnect. Like if I'm socializing with people, it's surface level, because it's like I'm wearing this mask, you know? I'll make superficial connections, but maybe that's it, you know?

Heather (therapist): So, you said there's a kind of disconnect and that when you're in these social situations you feel like you're wearing a mask. And it's just on the surface for you. (Thought Empathy: Chap. 4)

Kevin (patient): And it's even hard to make eye contact when I'm talking about this. The mask is off, you know, and if I make eye contact, it's uhh… Difficult to… Like, what are they seeing, you know?

Mike (therapist): As you were sharing that Kevin I felt kind of emotional. Like connecting with you and seeing your eyes welling up there a little bit. (I Feel Statements: Chap. 5) Some tears. Tell me, tell me what's happening there. (Inquiry: Chap. 5)

Kevin (patient): I guess it's… I'm not a very vulnerable person. And I feel embarrassed because everybody can see me.

Mike (therapist): It's hard to be vulnerable, isn't it? (Disarming: Chap. 4) Here we are in front of all these people who see those emotions coming out in the tears and feeling really embarrassed. (Feeling Empathy: Chap. 5) I wonder, I don't want to rush things along and it would be so beautiful to stay in this moment with you. I'd just love to hang out here for a while. (Chap. 5) At the same time, I wanted to check in with you, as to how Heather and I are doing at understanding what it's like for you right now. (Inquiry: Chap. 5)

Kevin (patient): Um, I'd give an "A minus." Yeah. I guess it's more me feeling like I'm holding back more.

Heather (therapist): So, you give us a pretty high score of an "A minus," but there's still something not quite fully connecting. And you notice that maybe you're holding back still a little bit. (Thought Empathy: Chap. 4) I'm wondering, in this moment, would you want to be fully seen and understood? (Inquiry: Chap. 5)

Kevin (patient): I think…. Yeah, I think I'm good with maybe maintaining a little bit because… I feel like maybe that was a bit of oversharing, like you know that's heavy for a lot of people and we also have a limited amount of time.

Heather (therapist): So, I think I hear you saying this is about as fully vulnerable and open as you'd want to be. (Thought Empathy: Chap. 4)

Kevin (patient): Yeah, yeah, I feel like, yeah, maintaining a little bit makes me feel more comfortable.

Mike (therapist): You kind of hinted also that there's a little bit of pressure on us, isn't there? (Feeling Empathy: Chap. 4)

Kevin (patient): Yeah. (*laughs*)

Mike (therapist): I am feeling that too! (I feel: Chap. 5) Can we just hang out and be pressured together? (Inquiry: Chap. 5)

Kevin (patient): OK, that sounds good. No problem.

Mike (therapist): I wonder if we, you know, made a little bit of a shift here into getting to work. Would now be an OK time to do that, or maybe there's more you would like to share? I don't want to rush into things. (Agenda Setting Step 1: Invitation: Chap. 6)

Kevin (patient): I guess there's also a part of me that thinks that if I open the gates up fully, that that would also be part of the overcompensation. Like, now I'm going into this character of oversharing and that's a bit much.

Heather (therapist): I just had this wave of admiration for you, Kevin. (Stroking: Chap. 5)

Mike (therapist): We could be just inauthentic for a while, or we could get to work? Agenda Setting Step 1: Invitation: Chap. 6)

Kevin (patient): (*laughing lightly*) That sounds good. Let's get to work.

Heather (therapist): So, I want to ask you, we've got about 50 minutes today, and just imagine that a miracle happens and you left here thinking that that was the most amazing session that could have possibly happened. What would be different? What would change? (*Note: Heather has delivered the Miracle Cure question which is not a skill covered in this training manual but can be used to obtain clarity of the patient's goals for therapy.*)

Kevin (patient): I guess I would feel totally authentic with myself.

Heather (therapist): If we were to ask why is that important to you, to be authentic with yourself? (Inquiry Chap. 5)

Kevin (patient): I guess I was always a shy, introverted kid. I switched schools a couple of times and I didn't really have many friends. So, I feel the mask kind of started coming in with, you know, trying desperately to connect to people, but I didn't really know how. So there were just a lot of shallow connections.

Heather (therapist): So, you're referring back to a time in school where you were shy, you'd move schools, and you desperately wanted to connect and make friends but didn't know how, and that's when the mask started. (Thought Empathy: Chap. 4)

Kevin (patient): And I also feel like the overcompensating or the over-extroverted personality, that it's kind of trying to make up for lost time or lost connections. It's like the introverted me. I can't really prioritize either one, because if I'm out socializing, I want to be by myself, but if I'm by myself, I feel like I should be socializing.

Mike (therapist): There is tension in the conflict there, isn't there? (Disarming: Chap. 4)

Kevin (patient): Yeah.

Mike (therapist): I was really feeling some of your, in a sense, loneliness and pain, when you shared. Moving schools reminded me of a time when I switched schools. Kind of felt like I had to be someone I wasn't. Just to survive. (I Feel: Chap. 5)

Kevin (patient): Yeah, and like just barely surviving.

Mike (therapist): Yeah. (Disarming: Chap. 4) Trying to keep your head above the water, but just enough to get a breath before you sink down again. (Thought Empathy: Chap. 4)

Kevin (patient): Yeah.

Mike (therapist): Well, I'm not entirely sure we can deliver your miracle cure.

Kevin (patient): Oh, that's a let down.

Mike (therapist): I would be wanting to offer you more than that. You said you'd like to feel totally authentic with yourself, and I'd be kind of hoping to offer that you feel amazing about yourself even when you're inauthentic. Would that be okay? (Pause) But you may not want that. (Addressing Process resistance: Dangling the Carrot: Chap. 11)

Kevin (patient): *(speaking to an audience member in the front row)* I was just looking out and I saw you welling up and that made me feel really emotional too. I can't really describe it all that much, but yeah. I also don't want to hold it up too much longer with me talking.

Mike (therapist): Kevin, we've done a little preparation before, and I wonder if it'd be OK for us to dive right in now. (Agenda Setting Step 1: Invitation: Chap. 6)

Kevin (patient): Yeah.

(Note: To save time in the demo we asked Kevin to fill out a blank Daily Mood Log (DML) prior to the session, pinpointing a moment in time when he was feeling upset and listing some of the emotions and thoughts in that moment. As Kevin's DML is being discussed, Mike and Heather have blank DML's of their own and they are filling them out as they go along.)

Mike (therapist): You prepared a daily mood log for us and you have pinpointed a moment in time where this experience that you're having this internal conflict occurred. (Agenda Step 2: Specificity: Chap. 7) And so I'm going to read through some of the things that you've written for the benefit of the audience. I also want to make sure we're really connecting with you as to what that experience is like and really help us to understand more deeply what it's like for you in those moments. So, Kevin, you noted here on the emotions that the upsetting event was at the end of lunch Friday at the conference by yourself. (Agenda Step 2: Specificity: Chap. 7)

Kevin (patient): Yeah.

Mike (therapist): And the emotions, the first one you circled was "unhappy," and it was 20% in the "Now" column. And then in the second column, you circled "worried" and "panicky" at 65, so fairly high. And then, "guilty" and "ashamed" you circled at 70. "Defective" and "incompetent" at 50 both. When you circled "rejected," rejecting of yourself, and you put that at 75. And then "embarrassed" and "self-conscious" at 60. And you mentioned before feeling kind of embarrassed even being up here. Has that increased or decreased? (Testing: Chap. 3 + Agenda Step 2: Specificity: Chap. 7)

Kevin (patient): It's increased a little right now, maybe 70.

Mike (therapist): OK, we'll just note that 70 on "embarrassing." And then "discouraged," just 20 and stuck at 40. And then the "other" column you wrote "overwhelmed" at 65. And you have done a beautiful job at identifying some of your negative thoughts already. The first one was "I should be socially on point all the time." And you put that 80% that you believe in right now. And then the second one is, "I'm a fraud. I'm inauthentic." And that was 95% true for you right now. The third negative thought: "People will see through my mask if I burn out." And that was 90%. And then number four, it was "People will think I'm awkward when I burnout," and that's at 95%. And the fifth one? "I'll miss out on possible connections if I don't socialize." And that was 100%. And then the other side of the page #6. "People might think I'm disinterested if I'm socially burnt out." That was 95. And just as we were sitting here, you wrote down another one. (Capturing & Refining Negative Thoughts: Chap. 13)

Kevin (patient): Yeah

Mike (therapist): Do you want to share that one? (Capturing & Refining Negative Thoughts: Chap. 13)

Kevin (patient): Sure. "People won't look at me the same after this."

Heather (therapist): And you scored that 100%. Thank you for laying this out also so beautifully, clearly. Are there any other thoughts? (Stroking: Chap. 5)

Kevin (patient): I think this is good. Yeah, my pleasure.

Heather (therapist): I noticed you circled "guilty" and "ashamed," that may be explained by these thoughts, but was there any other thought that was triggering that feeling? (Capturing & Refining Negative Thoughts: Chap. 13)

Kevin (patient): I guess there's that part of me that feels either guilty for burning out and having someone feel like I misled them, or that I don't care about the relationship when I do.

Heather (therapist): Can you phrase that in a statement that we might put on the daily mood log? (Capturing & Refining Negative Thoughts: Chap. 13)

Kevin (patient) Oh, sure, I guess maybe that goes with "the people might think that I'm disinterested if I'm burnt out and that I am inauthentic'. Yeah, there's a should. "I shouldn't let people down."

Heather (therapist): How much do you believe that thought? (Testing: Chap. 3)

Kevin (patient): 95.

Heather (therapist): Yeah, great. He's gonna write that down. I might just do one more pass at the Miracle Cure and say... Let's say we work on this and it's really transformational for you. What would you be hoping the change would be?

Kevin (patient): I guess... I wouldn't feel insecure. And I wouldn't need the mask. Not that I would become a total introvert and just throw the socializing away, but like, I wouldn't need that alternate version of myself to be socially outgoing.

Heather (therapist): Can I ask how insecure are you feeling right now? (Testing: Chap. 3)

Kevin (patient): Umm, maybe like a 70?

Heather (therapist): Can we write that under "overwhelmed" as another feeling? So now Kevin, imagine that we have a big red button right here. And if you push that button, that insecure feeling is just going to vanish. You're not going to have any of it at all. In fact, it's going to wipe away all these negative thoughts and feelings. Would you push that button? (Addressing Outcome Resistance: Magic Button Step 1: Chap. 9)

Kevin (patient): I'd push it to get rid of my insecurity. Yeah.

Heather (therapist): Great, so you send that insecurity down to zero. I'm excited because it sounds like you're really motivated. And at the same time, I'm a little bit hesitant. Because I'm thinking that your insecurity says a lot of pretty amazing things about you. Can we think about that together? (Addressing Outcome Resistance: Magic Button Step 2: Chap. 10)

Kevin (patient): Yes.

Heather (therapist): But what might possibly be positive about this feeling of insecurity? And we're going to go ahead and write that down. So can you pull out a blank piece of paper? And at the top we're going to write "Positive reframe." We're gonna do this together. Then you can draw a little column and a big column. The title of the little column is "thought or feeling." And the first feeling that we're going to positively reframe is the feeling of insecurity. So yeah, what comes to mind when you think of what could be positive about your capacity to feel insecure? (Addressing Outcome Resistance: Magic Button Step 2: Chap. 10)

Kevin (patient): I guess it's my wanting to be confident with myself.

Heather (therapist): Did you say wanting to be confident with yourself? What does that mean to you? Why is that important? (Addressing Outcome Resistance: Magic Button Step 2: Chap. 10)

Kevin (patient): I guess… I'm not really rejecting myself at that point.

Heather (therapist): And why is that important to you? To not reject yourself? (Addressing Outcome Resistance: Magic Button Step 2: Chap. 10)

Kevin (patient): Because I won't feel bad about myself…

Heather (therapist): I'm hearing the value of self-care, self-compassion. Is that right? Does it hurt to get rejected? (Addressing Outcome Resistance: Magic Button Step 2: Chap. 10)

Kevin (patient): Yeah.

Heather (therapist): And so, does it hurt if you reject yourself?

Kevin (patient): I think it hurts even more.

Heather (therapist): So, you're really wanting yourself not to suffer, not to have pain? (Addressing Outcome Resistance: Magic Button Step 2: Chap. 10)

Kevin (patient): Yeah.

Heather (therapist): Is that kind? (Addressing Outcome Resistance: Magic Button Step 2: Chap 10)

Kevin (patient): Yeah, I think so.

Heather (therapist): Is kindness important to you? (Addressing Outcome Resistance: Magic Button Step 2: Chap. 10)

Kevin (patient): Very important.

Heather (therapist): This feeling of insecurity, is it useful in any way? Does it serve any purpose that is helpful to you? (Addressing Outcome Resistance: Magic Button Step 2: Chap. 10)

Kevin (patient): I guess it's always kind of pushed me to try to figure out how to be a confident person. So, it's been behind my personal growth.

Heather (therapist): So, it's been really motivating. (Addressing Outcome Resistance: Magic Button Step 2: Chap. 10)

Kevin (patient): Yeah, yeah.

Heather (therapist): In any given moment when insecurity pops up, is that useful in any way? (Addressing Outcome Resistance: Magic Button Step 2: Chap. 10)

Kevin (patient): I think it tells me when I'm not being authentic.

Heather (therapist): Now remember… If you push that magic button it's going to completely wipe away your capacity to feel insecure. Would that be a problem for you at all? Like never feel insecure, ever. (Addressing Outcome Resistance: Magic Button Step 2: Chap. 10)

Kevin (patient): I think that would make me a sociopath.

Heather (therapist): So, there's something actually really important about your ability to feel insecure about it. That maybe relates to other people? When you said, "I'd be a sociopath if I could never feel insecure," can you say more? How does the capacity to feel insecure keep you from being a sociopath? (Addressing Outcome Resistance: Magic Button Step 2: Chap. 10)

Kevin (patient): I guess it kind of keeps the mask on.

Heather (therapist): So, it's actually connected to being true to yourself. (Addressing Outcome Resistance: Magic Button Step 2: Chap. 10)

Mike (therapist): I wonder too… This is just an idea, but you can tell me if it resonates. I wonder if it doesn't protect you in some way? Like if you become a social sociopath, how would people interact with you? (Addressing Outcome Resistance: Magic Button Step 2: Chap. 10)

Kevin (patient): I don't think people would want to be around me.

Mike (therapist): So, you are saying it protects you from rejection. Is that true? (Addressing Outcome Resistance: Magic Button Step 2: Chap. 10)

Kevin (patient): That's so ironic, so paradoxical.

Mike (therapist): Is it important, though? (Addressing Outcome Resistance: Magic Button Step 2: Chap. 10)

Kevin (patient): Yeah.

Heather (therapist): I mean, do you really believe that or are you just kind of going along with what we're saying? (Addressing Outcome Resistance: Magic Button Step 2: Chap. 10)

Kevin (patient): No, I think… Yeah. I mean, I'm not a psychologist, but if I was a sociopath, they wouldn't really care if people were rejecting them. So, if I lost the insecurity, then I guess I wouldn't really care about being rejected.

Mike (therapist): There is a solution. (Addressing Outcome Resistance: Magic Button Step 2: Chap. 10)

Heather (therapist): Yeah, is that a direction you'd like to go? (Addressing Outcome Resistance: Magic Button Step 2: Chap. 10)

Kevin (patient): No, not at all.

Mike (therapist): We just need to make you into a sociopath! (Addressing Outcome Resistance: Magic Button Step 2: Chap. 10)

Kevin (patient): No, no. Because then, if I was a sociopath, then I wouldn't know if I was hurting, or I wouldn't care if I was hurting anybody.

Mike (therapist): Sounds great.

Heather (therapist): Are you saying that you care if you hurt other people? So your insecurity is connected to really caring about other people as well as yourself. (Addressing Outcome Resistance: Magic Button Step 2: Chap. 10) What I would suggest to you for homework, Kevin, is that you go through, and you positively reframe each emotion. Normally I would spend a little more time doing one or two others, and then assign the rest as homework. (Assigning Homework: Chap. 17)

Mike (therapist): Kevin, we've got 10 or 11 really wonderful reasons for you to continue feeling insecure. Maybe it would be better if Heather and I helped you to feel more insecure with all these wonderful benefits. (Addressing Outcome Resistance: Magic Button Step 2: Chap. 10)

Kevin (patient): I don't know... I'm... I'm kind of tired of rejecting myself all the time.

Mike (therapist): It's painful, isn't it? Yeah. We have this kind of dilemma on our hands, don't we? On the one hand, it's painful to be rejecting yourself and feel that insecurity. On the other hand, we have all these wonderful benefits, and it really shows some amazing things about your values and your character. What if, instead of a magic button, Heather and I offered you a magic dial, where we could dial down your insecurity to just the right amount? We don't know the sweet spot where we retain all these benefits but not have it be so painful. How does that sound? (Addressing Outcome Resistance: Magic Button Step 2: Chap. 10)

Kevin (patient): That sounds perfect.

(Note: Kevin goes on to set goals for each feeling on a scale of 0-100: Insecure 20, Unhappy 15, Guilty & Ashamed 5, Defective 15, Rejected 5, Embarrassed 5, Discouraged 2, Stuck 2, Overwhelmed 5.)

Mike (therapist): I love your goals here, and I think we can hit those. But I do have a warning for you. There's no guarantees. But some of these tools are very powerful. And we may overshoot. You might end up feeling less than 15% defective. And if that happens, I can show you how to be more defective. Will that be okay? (Addressing Process Resistance: Dangling the Carrot: Chap. 11)

Kevin (patient): That will be okay.

Heather (therapist): Kevin, we've just finished agenda setting and we're ready to move on to methods. I'm wondering how insecure you're feeling right now?

Kevin (patient): About the same. But anxiety definitely spiked when you said "methods." *(laughs)*

Heather (therapist): Yes. OK. So, what we would suggest is we start with one thought, and we'll see if we can make some shift with that thought. Usually if one thought tumbles, the rest tend to go. (Addressing Process Resistance: Dangling the Carrot: Chap. 11) So is there a thought here you'd like to start with?

Kevin (patient): Number 7.

Heather (therapist): Number 7: "People won't see me the same way after this." Kevin, you have some familiarity with TEAM. Is there a method you would like us to do?

(Note: At this point, we would create what is called a "recovery circle," and we would choose from a variety of methods and fail as fast as we can to find the right one. When we are working with patients, we ask them to help us come up with the recovery circle based on the reading they've been doing in the homework because they have insights we do not have, and we have insights they do not have. And together, we combine and develop a super powerful treatment plan.)

Kevin (patient): Though it makes me anxious and nervous, I think exposure would probably be it.

Heather (therapist): So, you mentioned exposure and exposure is most effective when we go at the core fear. (Addressing Process Resistance: Dangling the Carrot: Chap. 11) We will definitely include that as part of our treatment plan today and for homework. So, there's also a technique called "externalization of voices." Mike is going to explain it.

Mike (therapist): In externalization of voices, I'm Kevin. I'm you. But I'm your negative thoughts. And I'm gonna attack you with your negative thoughts and your job is to defeat me. To argue back. To crush me. (Methods: Externalization of Voices: Chap. 14) There are three ways you can do that. First is by defending yourself and arguing, saying "no, that's not true and here's why." The second is through accepting it with a sense of humor and grace and self-compassion and that it doesn't bother you at all. The third is what we call "counterattack." And that's where you talk back to the negative voice itself. Regardless of the content of the negative thought, you just dismiss it. And if we get stuck, we can roll, reverse, and I can model alternate options for you to try out. Ready? (How to Defeat Negative Thoughts: Chap. 15)

Kevin (patient): Yeah.

Mike (therapist): Who am I?

Kevin (patient): You're my negative thoughts.

Mike (therapist): And who are you?

Kevin (patient): I'm the positive Kevin.

Mike (therapist): Yeah. Kevin, can I speak with you for a moment? (Externalization of Voices: Chap. 14)

Kevin (patient): I'd rather not. (*laughs*) Yeah, go ahead.

Mike (therapist): What just happened right there?

Kevin (patient): I guess… I just shoved it away or kind of rejected the rejection.

Mike (therapist): Who is winning? Negative Kevin or positive Kevin? (Externalization of Voices: Chap. 14)

Kevin (patient): Positive, I think positive Kevin.

Mike (therapist): Was it a small win or a big win? (Externalization of Voices: Chap. 14)

Kevin (patient): I think it was big.

Mike (therapist): What was it huge? (Externalization of Voices: Chap. 14)

Kevin (patient): Let's keep it at big.

Mike (therapist): So, Kevin, I'm that negative voice in your head. And I just wanna remind you, you know, you're at that conference and feeling kind of burnt out with all the socializing and everything. And really, you're an introvert and you're exhausted and overwhelmed. And I just wanted to let you know that people see you burned out and they won't look at you the same way. I don't want you to feel bad, but just "people are not gonna look at you the same." (Externalization of Voices: Chap. 14)

Kevin (patient): Yeah, you're right! *(laughs)*

Mike (therapist): Who's winning right now, positive Kevin or negative? (Externalization of Voices: Chap. 14)

Kevin (patient): I think I am.

Mike (therapist): Yeah. Small or big? (Externalization of Voices: Chap. 14)

Kevin (patient): I think that was big.

Mike (therapist): Huge? (Externalization of Voices: Chap. 14)

Kevin (patient): Yeah, I think that was pretty huge.

Mike (therapist): And how did you win? (Processing Learning: Chap. 16)

Kevin (patient): I just accepted it.

Mike (therapist) For humor's sake, you wanna do a little role reversal?

Kevin (patient): Yeah!

Mike (therapist): I can show you a couple of alternate ways. (How to Defeat Negative Thoughts: Chap. 15)

Kevin (patient): OK.

Mike (therapist): Also, for a bit of a teaching point: Now, before I dive into this and if he wins huge, I would say, "OK, let's write that down. What did you say?" In fact, we could probably do that right now. Yeah, let's write that down. What was your Positive thought? (Processing Learning: Chap. 16)

Kevin (patient): "I think you're right."

Mike (therapist): So that was the acceptance.

Kevin (patient): Yeah.

Mike (therapist): Let's do a quick roll reversal. So, you become "negative Kevin," I'll be positive and I'll model for you each of the three options. And then you can decide whether you want to add any of those pieces in when we switch back. (How to Defeat Negative Thoughts: Chap. 15)

Kevin (patient): [*As negative Kevin*] Hey, I just wanted to let you know that, you know, you were really kind of oversharing a little bit. People now see through your facade, and they think that you're fake and they won't look at you the same.

Mike (therapist): [*As positive Kevin*] Well, I have a couple of responses to that. The first is that's just a load of crap because this is a room of really caring and loving therapists, arguably the nicest place in the world to be right now. so I don't buy your BS. The second thing is, that's actually the best thing that can happen. I don't want people to look at me the same anymore. I wanna see them see me as

I really am. The best fraud ever! (How to Defeat Negative Thoughts: Chap. 15) Who is winning right now? (Processing Learning: Chap. 16)

Kevin (patient): That was huge.

Mike (therapist): And what resonated with you? (Processing Learning: Chap. 16)

Kevin (patient): I think when you mentioned that I'm in a room of therapists. That it really sounded ridiculous that by talking about my feelings I would get judged. And I felt really safe when you said that.

Heather (therapist): [*As negative Kevin*] Hey, Kevin. (Externalization of Voices: Chap. 14)

Kevin (patient): Hey.

Heather (therapist): I'm back. (Externalization of Voices: Chap. 14)

Kevin (patient): Welcome. [*laughs*]

Heather (therapist): OK, we have 3 minutes, this is a flash round. "People are never gonna see you the same again after this" (Externalization of Voices: Chap. 14)

Kevin (patient): Yeah. I think you're right. I've been kind of wearing this mask for a while and it's getting pretty heavy, and you know, I kind of want to let that go and let people see me.

Heather (therapist): And who won that? (Processing Learning: Chap. 16)

Kevin (patient): I did!

Heather (therapist) Big or Small? (Processing Learning: Chap. 16)

Kevin (patient) Big.

Heather (therapist) Big or huge? (Processing Learning: Chap. 16)

Kevin (patient) Huge.

(Note: At this point, we added one more method called "rejection practice," which is not covered in this book.)

Mike (therapist): Let's do one really high-speed exposure, OK? All of these people here are gonna be the "therapists from hell." And they're judgmental and mean. So, we're gonna do a group rejection. Are you ready for this?

Kevin (patient): I hope so.

Mike (therapist): I want you to ask them the question, "What do you think of me right now?"

And all of you in the audience, your answer is "we reject you and look down on you right now!" Are you ready for this, Kevin?

Kevin (patient): Okay.

Mike (therapist): And you have to look them in the eye.

Kevin (patient): I'm a little anxious.

Mike (therapist): How anxious?

Kevin (patient): Uh, let's say 8 out of 10.

Mike (therapist): OK, beautiful. Good. Remember, look them in the eye.

Kevin (patient): Like in individual people or everyone as a group?

Mike (therapist): You are going to scan the group, they're all gonna look right in your eyes.

Kevin (patient): And what am I asking?

Mike (therapist): "What do you think of me right now?". And they're all gonna reject you at the same time.

Kevin (patient): OK. [*To the audience*] What do you guys think of me right now?

Group together: "We reject you!"

Mike (therapist): How does that feel? (Processing Learning: Chap. 16)

Kevin (patient): More like a 6 out of 10.

Mike (therapist) OK. Let's do it one more time.

Kevin (patient): [*To the audience*] So I was just wondering how you guys are all looking at me right now. What do you guys think?

Group together: "We reject you!"

Kevin (patient): I don't believe you. Not all.

Heather (therapist): And so what's your anxiety level right now? (Processing Learning: Chap. 16)

Kevin (patient): Like a 3.

Heather (therapist): And how insecure are you feeling right now? (Testing: Chap. 3)

Kevin (patient): Like literally, I'm not really insecure at all.

Heather (therapist): Did we go too low?

Kevin (patient): Maybe like 10%.

Mike (therapist): You are not a sociopath now, are you? (*laughs*)

Kevin (patient): I don't know, yeah, I don't think so. (*laughs*)

Heather (therapist): Great! Now we've got some homework for you. (Assigning Homework: Chap. 17)

Kevin (patient): OK.

Heather (therapist): The first would be to fill out your mood scores afterwards so you can see the impact of what we've done. We'd like you to fill out the 'brief mood survey' and the 'evaluation of therapy' form. (Testing: Chap. 3) And then we were thinking that you might do some more exposure by individually asking about 20 people in the room what they think of you. (Assigning Homework: Chap. 17)

Kevin (patient) Really, after this?

Heather (therapist): [*Speaking to the audience members*] And your job is, if Kevin asks you, to be completely honest. Yeah, if you feel judgmental, you should let him know that. And if you feel warm and caring, you could let him know that too. (Assigning Homework: Chap. 17)

Kevin (patient): Oh. Thank you so much!

Audience claps and gives Kevin a standing ovation.

Kevin (patient): Oh, that's too much. Sit down. OK, cut it out! (*laughs*)

Chapter 19
Conclusion: We Never "Arrive": A Lifelong Commitment Toward Better Patient Outcomes

One of the first things you will hear when you come into a TEAM-CBT training group is the request to "check your ego at the door" and "fail as fast as you can." These two statements are meant to underscore the approach of learning through feedback and successive refinement. The idea is that we can improve patient outcomes if we accept responsibility for our part in making therapy better.

Sir David John Brailsford, the coach of the UK cycling team, led the previously underwhelming team to unprecedented achievements in the cycling world. His approach: commitment to excellence in every aspect. Not only in strength, endurance, and technique, but also working on continuous incremental improvements in their nutrition, gear, hydration, and lifestyle. A famous example of his approach is his insistence that the hotels in which the cycling pros stay during and before competitions have particular mattresses to improve their night sleep. The team would travel with a trailer stacked with mattresses that would be hauled each night into the athlete's rooms on the road (Moore, 2014). The lesson is that there is no quick, easy way toward superior professional outcomes. Each *incremental* improvement wins the race.

This book focuses on the key therapy skills TEAM-CBT offers for improved therapy processes, workflows, and outcomes. We encourage you to apply the same approach of continuous refinement to all professional skills – those practiced inside *and* outside the therapy room. This may include going beyond "therapy" skills and getting better at skills such as explaining your therapy approach to patients and colleagues, better clinical note taking, better billing practices, better response to phone inquiries, better video experience for teletherapy, better communication, better homework assignments, etc. All these incremental improvements enhance the quality of services and, yes, better patient outcomes.

If there is one message we want to drive home on this closing note, it is that the commitment to engage in incremental improvements is a *lifelong* process with no clear end state. Indeed, one of the best predictors of therapist effects is a humble attitude toward continuous learning. Humbly accepting that we can always improve,

M. Katz et al., *Deliberate Practice of TEAM-CBT*, SpringerBriefs in Psychology, https://doi.org/10.1007/978-3-031-46019-7_19

we assume that to be a psychotherapy expert means, curiously enough, to never arrive at total expertise! In our training groups, we often refer to it as "joyous failure." A prominent psychotherapy researcher, Helene Nissen-Lie, recently summarized this in the form of a rather poetic advice: "Love yourself as a person, doubt yourself as a therapist" (Nissen-Lie et al., 2017).

We hope that this book will keep exciting and challenging you to engage in this lifelong adventure. With the help of motivated supervisors and peers, we urge you to set a high bar for yourself and your own professional development – to keep monitoring your outcomes, asking for feedback whenever possible, and engaging in deliberate practice to incrementally help more patients, more often. We salute your efforts and thank you for letting us be part of your journey!

References

Moore, R. (2014). *Mastermind: How Dave Brailsford Reinvented the Wheel*. BackPage Press.

Nissen-Lie, H. A., Rønnestad, M. H., Høglend, P. A., Havik, O. E., Solbakken, O. A., Stiles, T. C., & Monsen, J. T. (2017). Love yourself as a person, doubt yourself as a therapist? *Clinical Psychology & Psychotherapy, 24*(1), 48–60.

Index